J. Thomas Danzi, M.D., is the chief
of gastroenterology at the Guthrie
Clinic in Sayre, Pennsylvania. He has
written numerous articles on
digestive diseases in leading medical
journals.

J. THOMAS DANZI, M.D., F.A.C.P.

Free Yourself from Digestive Pain

A Guide to Preventing and Curing Your Digestive Illness

PRENTICE HALL PRESS · NEW YORK

Published in 1987 by Prentice Hall Press
A Division of Simon & Schuster, Inc.
Gulf + Western Building
One Gulf + Western Plaza
New York, NY 10023

Originally published by Prentice-Hall, Inc.

PRENTICE HALL PRESS is a trademark of Simon & Schuster, Inc.

Library of Congress Cataloging-in-Publication Data
Danzi, J. Thomas.
    Free yourself from digestive pain.

    Bibliography: p.
    Includes index.
    1. Digestive organs—Diseases—Psychosomatic aspects.
2. Stress (Physiology)   3. Abdominal pain.   I. Title.
RC806.D36 1984   616.3   83-24410
ISBN 0-13-330663-1 (pbk.)

Manufactured in the United States of America

10   9   8   7   6   5   4   3   2

First Prentice Hall Press Edition

Contents

Preface

The human digestive system is responsible for more human suffering than any other body organ system. All of us, at one time or another, have known the heartbreak of acid indigestion, the consequence of bowel irregularity, the plight of hemorrhoidal pain, or the social embarrassment of excess intestinal gas.

Recent data collected by a national advisory board on digestive disease estimates that half of the American population suffers intermittently with digestive dysfunction. It is known that more than 20 million Americans suffer with gallbladder disease and more than 4 million Americans have peptic ulcer disease. Hundreds of millions of people have either hemorrhoidal problems or tension-related digestive disorders.

The cost to all of us for relief of digestive diseases is astronomical and increasing yearly. Americans spend approximately $150 million annually on nonprescription antacids and "over-the-counter" bowel regulators. The final annual bill for the treatment of all digestive diseases, including hospitalizations, operations, and medications is approximately $20 million.

Why are digestive diseases so common? One reason is that the digestive system is very susceptible to stress and tension. Tension plays an important role in causing stomach upset, the spastic colon syndrome, and belly pain. Tobacco, alcohol, coffee, and aspirin are common substances used habitually to reduce our daily tension. Unfortunately, all these substances are detrimental to the normal functioning of the digestive system.

This book will review various maladies of the digestive system and, I hope, help in the understanding of the gut feelings that result from its abnormal function.

I wish to acknowledge Mrs. Darlene Updyke for her transcriptional assistance and Mrs. Rosamarie Hadlock for the preparation of the illustrations.

This book is dedicated to my father, who lost his life as a result of severe peptic ulcer disease.

The writing of this book was possible because of the understanding and cooperation of my wife and family.

chapter one

Acid Indigestion
or the Stressful Stomach

All of us have experienced the sensation of acid indigestion, that burning, gnawing sensation in the pit of our stomachs. Some experience it regularly and some only on special occasions.

Why do we experience acid indigestion? To understand the answer to this question, we must first appreciate the normal anatomy and function of the stomach.

How the Stomach Functions

Food enters the stomach after passing from the mouth into the gullet (food tube), or esophagus as it is known medically. While the injested food is in the stomach, the digestive process begins so the body can take up or absorb the food's important constituents. The food stimulates the stomach to produce digestive juices, or enzymes, and acid that enters into the stomach cavity. The acid is necessary for the proper functioning of the digestive juices. The food is then propelled by the stomach's movements or peristalsis into the first portion of the small intestine known as the duodenum. Here, in the small intestines, the majority of the digestive process takes place.

Some medical experts have referred to the stomach as a pouch full of acid, namely, hydrochloric acid. We all know that acid is corrosive and will eat through various metals if in strong enough concentration. Why then does the stomach not digest itself since it is full of acid? We have all heard the phrase "he has a cast-iron stomach." It is also true that there are trace amounts of minerals, such as iron, that are important to the daily functioning of our body. However, the iron concentration is not significant enough to form a barrier within the stomach and is not the reason that the stomach does not digest itself.

There is a sophisticated pumping mechanism contained within the stomach's lining that prevents the acid from reentering the stomach in strong enough concentration to do any harm.[1] This pumping mechanism works very efficiently unless the stomach lining is damaged. Gastritis is the medical name for an inflamed or injured stomach lining. Only when gastritis is present can a sufficient amount of acid reenter the stomach lining and cause ulcerations to occur. Gastritis will be further described in Chapter 2.

Stomach pains, the classic stomachache, is different from acid indigestion. Belly aches, that full feeling, result most commonly from dietary indiscretions or the consumption of culinary delights beyond a sensible limit. All of us have experienced that full turkey feeling after a large Thanksgiving Day meal, important business dinners, or drinking too much fluid after vigorous exercise. This sensation usually resolves, with time, as the quantity of food or liquid passes from the stomach into the beginning of the small intestine.

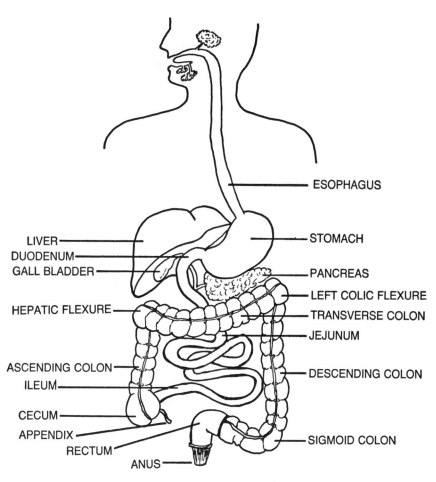

ESOPHAGUS

LIVER
DUODENUM
GALL BLADDER

STOMACH

PANCREAS
LEFT COLIC FLEXURE

HEPATIC FLEXURE

TRANSVERSE COLON
JEJUNUM

ASCENDING COLON
ILEUM

DESCENDING COLON

CECUM
APPENDIX
RECTUM
ANUS

SIGMOID COLON

ILLUSTRATION 1. Digestive system.

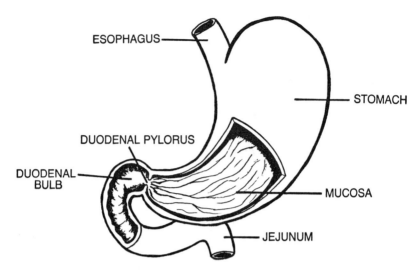

ESOPHAGUS

STOMACH

DUODENAL PYLORUS

DUODENAL BULB

MUCOSA

JEJUNUM

ILLUSTRATION 2. The Upper Digestive Tract.

There is an important difference among individuals' tolerance for specific foods. It is clear that certain foods are not tolerated by specific individuals. The cause for this intolerance is not fully understood; however, in the majority of cases it is not shown to be due to a food allergy or a specific disease state of the digestive tract.

Causes of Acid Indigestion

Acid indigestion does not seem to be related to what you eat, but rather to what is eating you. Stressful situations resulting from anger, fear, frustrations, and anxiety have a dramatic effect on the stomach's function. During times of stress the stomach is acted upon by the vagus nerve.[2] This nerve has an important role in preparing the body for response to the situation. This response is known as the flight or fight reaction. We are prepared to respond to the stressful situation both internally and externally. We can all remember our feelings when startled at night or having to react to an emergency situation. Our heightened reactions, the awareness of our heart beating rapidly within our chest and the "pins and needles" sensation of our skin. All of these physical signs are the result of the preparation for our body to respond from the signals it has received from our nervous system. In times of stress, the stomach lining becomes as red and mad as we feel. In response to the vagal nerve stimulation, the stomach pours out large amounts of digestive juices and acid.[3] The stomach's movements or contractions are also increased as a result of this stimulation. The combination of both the increased secretions and motility can clearly result in acid indigestion.

Stress, besides the previously mentioned effects on the function of the stomach, may cause belly pain due to air swallowing. Aerophagia, the act of regular air swallowing, results most commonly as a result of chronic anxiety or stress. The consumed air distends the stomach and causes pain with continuous belching. It has been said, "people swallow air who cannot swallow life."[4] In times of acute stress, some of us may swallow enough air to compound the coexisting acid indigestion. A further discussion of air swallowing, or aerophagia, will be forthcoming in the chapter relating to intestinal gas.

Unfortunately, stressful situations also dictate many of our social habits. We do things to help decrease the stress we are under and make our life more tolerable. Smoking, alcoholic consumption, coffee drinking, and aspirin ingestion are all common means by which people relax. Unfortunately, all of these have been shown to have a detrimental effect on the stomach.[5,6] These commonly practiced social habits are all associated with either an increased production of stomach acid or the ability to predispose the stomach lining to either chronic or acute inflammation. Therefore, the means that we use to reduce life's stresses predispose us to acid indigestion.

Aspirin ingestion, for the relief of tension headaches, is one of the most commonly practiced routines in America. Detailed scientific research has clearly shown that aspirin ingestion can cause gastritis or stomach lining inflammation, bleeding from the stomach lining, and ulcerations of the stomach.[7,8] The bleeding from the stomach, which is the result of the regular high-dose usage of aspirin, may produce either a rapid or slow bleeding state from the stomach lining. A slow bleeding condition of the stomach lining would result in the continual loss of iron, contained within the red blood cells, from the body. This would gradually result in an anemia with the resultant symptoms of malaise and easy fatigability. More importantly, aspirin ingestion could result in a state of brisk bleeding from the lining of the stomach. In this situation the individual may vomit bright red blood or dark blood looking like coffee-ground material. They may either pass dark black-colored stools or pass bright red blood per rectum. A further discussion of the various symptoms of bleeding from the stomach or upper portion of the small intestine will be discussed in Chapter 2.

Most commonly, most sufferers of acid indigestion use antacids for relief. Antacids are usually effective in relieving acid indigestion. However, if our social habits are persistent or our stressful situations are unchanged, persistent acid indigestion will not be relieved by the antacids. The intermittent use of antacids for acid indigestion is acceptable. However, if the acid indigestion becomes persistent or if the burning pain in the pit of the stomach awakens us from sleep at night, medical advice should be sought to exclude the presence of an active peptic ulcer. The antacids render their effect by coating the lining of the stomach and by decreasing the concentration of acid within the stomach. In Chapter 2 a detailed discussion of antacids will be presented. Information to help in the selection of an antacid, the risk involved with the abuse of antacids, and the proper method to take antacids will be discussed. The question of whether these commonly used drugs are always safe will also be answered.

The stomach reacts as we do to our environment. Stressful situations dramatically affect the stomach's function. Acid indigestion is one of the many symptoms that can result as a consequence of that interaction. Our daily encounters have more important and meaningful effects on us than do encounters of the third kind.

chapter two

Peptic Ulcer Disease

Peptic ulcer disease affects more than 4 million Americans. This affliction has a dramatic effect on these individuals' life styles and a great economic impact on both the country and individuals. The fiscal reality of ulcer disease becomes evident when one realizes the cost of the care of those 4 million people is close to $4 billion annually. In addition, they spend close to $150 million yearly on the purchase of antacids for pain relief. More importantly, in 1977 for example, earnings lost by patients with ulcer disease amounted to $680 million. It becomes evident what a devastating illness simple ulcer disease is.

I bring tidings of good news. The incidence of occurrence of peptic ulcer disease has been decreasing in recent years. Both stomach ulcers and duodenal ulcers, an ulceration in the first portion of the small intestine, are being recognized less frequently.[1] The reason why fewer Americans are developing peptic ulcers remains unknown to digestive disease experts. It is known that a significant decrease has occurred in the rate in which men are being diagnosed with new duodenal ulcers. Duodenal ulcers still occur more frequently in males than females. However, instead of the former 9 to 1 ratio, the ratio is now 2 to 1. Both men and women develop stomach ulcers at an equal rate of occurrence.

Women may be paying for their recent socioeconomic advances. It was in the mid-1970s, coincidental with major change in the female employment pattern, that women were recognized to have duodenal ulcers at an increased rate. More women were working full time and in high-pressure positions. Does this bit of information illustrate the detrimental effect of stress on the digestive system? Does the tension of our jobs lead to peptic ulcer disease? Before answering those questions, I would like to discuss what a peptic ulcer is.

What a Peptic Ulcer Is

An ulcer is an open sore on the lining of the stomach or duodenum. Peptic means the association with gastric acid or the hydrochloric acid produced by the stomach to aid in the digestive process. Therefore, a peptic ulcer results from the effect of acid on the lining of stomach or duodenum. It all seems simple to understand. Ulcer disease has been recognized from the time of the ancient Egyptians. Yet today, digestive disease experts cannot explain adequately why some individuals with excess stomach acid develop ulcerations and others do not.[2]

It is known that individuals with duodenal ulcers are typically hypersecretors of stomach acid.[3] That is, they produce an increased amount of acid to varying stimulants such as foods, alcohol, and coffee. The amount of stomach acid a person with a duodenal ulcer may produce after a meal may vary from two to five times the amount normally secreted. However, the exact mechanism by which this excess acid in the beginning of the small intestine causes an ulcer remains to be determined by our research colleague. The majority of people with stomach ulcers are similar to their duodenal ulcer counterparts in that they secrete more acid than normal. However, some stomach ulcer patients make less than normal amounts of hydrochloric acid in response to various stimulants. The low level of acid output in these individuals is the result of a chronic inflammation of the stomach lining known as a chronic gastritis. This chronic gastritis can result from the natural aging process or from the habitual ingestion of materials known to be harmful to the stomach lining. Alcoholic beverages and aspirin containing compounds are the two most commonly recognized causes of chronic gastritis. If then some individuals with stomach ulcers produce below-normal amounts of stomach acid, why do they develop the ulcerations? The gastritis causes the ulcers to occur in the inflamed stomach lining; these ulcers are not caused by acid, as are duodenal ulcers.

The Effect of Stress

It becomes evident that there is no common denominator among individuals with peptic ulcer disease except for the increased acid production. What then is the possible relationship between stress or anxiety and the development of ulcer disease? It is well known that stressful situations result in an increase in stomach acid output. This increased acid production is the consequence of the greater than normal nervous stimulation to the stomach lining. It would seem obvious then that prolonged periods of heightened tension or anxiety would lead to an observed increase in peptic ulcer disease. This is not the case, however. There appears to be need for another factor besides the excess acid. In most individuals there is a protective substance that shields the digestive organs' lining from the development of ulcerations. Only in those people who have a decreased amount of this protective substance and excess stomach acid will peptic ulcers occur. I am sorry to say it is not our jobs that cause ulcers. It is partly our own fault.

Symptoms of a Peptic Ulcer

What are the signs that might indicate that an individual has an active peptic ulcer? Duodenal and stomach ulcerations cause slightly different symptoms in those afflicted with them. Duodenal ulcer patients usually notice a gnawing or deep hurting sensation in the pit of their stomachs. This feeling has sometimes been described as a severe hunger pain located between the rib cages and below the bottom of the breast bone. This sensation most commonly occurs thirty minutes to an hour after eating. This would coincide with the time that the stomach acid production is at its highest point. This acid, on the open sore in the lining of the duodenum, causes pain similar to that which vinegar, a weak acid, would cause on an open sore of the fingers or hand. Another feature of duodenal ulcer pain is that antacids or milk or a small snack will typically relieve the discomfort in a couple of minutes.

A similar gnawing or hurting sensation may awaken people with duodenal ulcers in the middle of the night. This nocturnal pain is experienced by many individuals with an active duodenal ulcer. This nighttime pain is usually associated with deeper ulcerations of the duodenum.

As previously mentioned, stomach ulcers produce different symptoms than those occurring in people with duodenal ulcerations. The classic "food-pain" cycle, observed with ulcers of the duodenum, is less commonly observed in individuals with stomach ulcerations. The pain may have no relationship to eating or it may occur later than an hour after meals. However, the discomfort is again described as a deep hurt or gnawing sensation in the pit of the stomach. An important distinguishing feature of gastric ulcer pain is the nonpredictability of antacids or food to relieve this discomfort.

Both stomach and duodenal ulcers have a seasonal occurrence. Both types of ulcerations occur more frequently in the spring and fall of the year. Most complications of peptic ulcer disease, especially bleeding from ulcers, seem to occur more frequently during those two seasons. Digestive disease experts have no readily available explanation for these observations. Could concern about tax preparation and the April 15th deadline somehow be related to the spring occurrence of ulcer disease? Is it the tension of the Monday-night football games or the domestic consequence of all the football games that are implicated with the fall increase? It will take carefully planned long-term studies to accurately delineate the reasons.

There is a common saying in the medical field regarding peptic ulcer disease: "Once an ulcer, always an ulcer." What does this mean exactly? Certainly ulcerations heal, but duodenal ulcers, more than stomach ulcers, have a tendency to recur.[4,5] The observed high recurrence rate with duodenal ulcers is most likely related to the persistence of predisposing factors. This means that individuals with a history of an ulceration in the duodenum will commonly have a sensitive stomach with a lot of heartburn and acid indigestion symptoms between documented occurrences of their ulceration.

It is important that you do not label yourself as an ulcer patient without proper medical evaluation. Most people with acid indigestion or stomach pain will be shown not to have a peptic ulcer as the source of their symptoms. If you think that you may have an ulcer, seek medical advice.

Diagnosis of Peptic Ulcers

What will this usually entail? In the majority of cases the physician will be able to diagnose peptic ulcer disease from the history of your symptoms, the findings of the physical examination, and the results of the upper GI X-ray test. The upper GI X-ray is also known as a barium swallow, which is accomplished after an overnight fast. In some cases the physician might not obtain an X-ray if the history and physical findings are typical of ulcer disease. Once an ulcer is diagnosed, proper medical therapy should alleviate the symptoms within seven to ten days unless a complication has occurred. A complete discussion of the therapy of peptic ulcer disease will be accomplished later in this chapter.

Sometimes this initial evaluation will not document an ulceration in an individual who the physician feels has a definite ulcer. Probably 10 percent of cases with active peptic ulcer disease are not correctly diagnosed with the conventional radiology examination.[6] In this circumstance the physician may elect to treat and observe for a response to the therapy or may request an endoscopic examination of the upper digestive tract to be performed. An endoscopic exam is also known as an upper GI endoscopy or gastroduodenoscopy. What does this examination entail and why would it be done?

After an overnight fast, a flexible instrument, or endoscope, is passed through the mouth down into the gullet, stomach, and duodenum. This endoscope has controls that enable the physician to carefully steer and control the passage of the instrument. This instrument enables the doctor to examine the lining of those organs directly with his eyesight and determine if an ulceration is present. Photographs and tissue samples or biopsies could be obtained with this endoscope if the physician felt they were necessary. Prior to such an examination, the patient would have the back of his or her throat numbed or anesthetized with a novacaine-like spray or drink. This preparation enables the person to swallow the instrument more easily. Sometimes patients will be given drugs intravenously to sedate them during the procedure. The use of the sedative medication will vary among doctors' practice characteristics and the person's apprehension regarding the test. The important facts regarding upper GI endoscopy is that it is safe and 98 percent accurate in diagnosing peptic ulcer disease.[7]

A very important point to remember is that all duodenal ulcers are benign; that is, nonmalignant. However,
about 25 percent of stomach ulcers are malignant. These malignant stomach ulcers do not arise from benign stomach ulcerations but are an ulcer within a stomach cancer. All patients with an ulceration of the stomach must be carefully
followed to demonstrate complete healing of the ulcer.[8] This
follow-up is necessary because most malignant ulcerations of
the stomach will not heal completely. Therefore, once a
stomach ulcer is diagnosed, your doctor will want you to have
repeat upper GI X-ray tests or to have an endoscopic examination so that tissue samples may be analyzed to exclude the
presence of a cancer.

Treatment for Ulcer Disease

What is the treatment of ulcer disease? What is the role of
diet in the therapy for peptic ulcer disease? What about all
these new ulcer miracle drugs? There has been a dramatic
change in the treatment of peptic ulcer disease within the last
decade. Formerly there was a great concern about the role of
the diet in the treatment of individuals with ulcers. Patients
were treated with various bland diets or milk-products-only
diets while their ulcers were causing stymptoms and for
sometime after the ulcerations had healed. Today most digestive disease experts believe that dietary changes have no
proven benefit in the healing of active peptic ulcerations.[9]
Most doctors allow their patients with ulcer disease to eat
whatever they can tolerate and advise them to avoid only
those foods that upset their stomachs. Even today some of
my patients with ulcer disease will only eat a bland diet when
having active symptoms. In discussing this they say this tendency is mostly out of habit. I would recommend that individuals with ulcer disease try to liberalize their diets. Learn what
you can and cannot tolerate. It will certainly make the cook's
job a lot easier, and individuals with ulcers will probably be
surprised by the good foods they will be able to enjoy.
    The most important part of the treatment of ulcer

disease has always been the reduction of the excess stomach acid.[10] This has been accomplished by the use of antacids alone or in combination with drugs that are designed for this purpose. Let's discuss antacids first. There are a myriad of over-the-counter antacid preparations available today. They vary in their color, taste, and price. Importantly they are different in the composition of their active ingredients. Some antacids contain various carbonate salts; others are comprised of aluminum hydroxide; and others contain various magnesium compounds. One, Pepto-Bismol, has bismuth subsalicylate as its main ingredient. Simethicone, an antigas or bubble reducer, is added to some of the antacid preparations. More importantly these various antacids vary considerably in their ability to neutralize or reduce stomach acid. That is correct, folks. All antacids are not created equal. How should you choose which one to use?

Choosing an Antacid

I tell my patients to select an antacid preparation with the taste they like and would be willing to take regularly. If they cannot swallow the antacid, it certainly will not be helping to heal their ulcer. I have no preference toward antacids that contain or do not contain simethicone. Again, if individuals notice a difference, I would recommend their preferred antacids for their usage.

How often you take your antacid will depend upon your doctor's opinion and your symptoms. Most physicians will recommend to their patients with ulcer disease that they take their antacid one hour after meals to allow the antacid to buffer the stomach acid, which is produced in its greatest quantity at that time. Your doctor will probably suggest a dose of antacid before retiring at bedtime so the preparation can protect the ulcer during the night. Initially the frequency of antacid usage may be increased until the ulcer pain disappears. This might mean that you would be taking the antacid hourly or every two hours. Once the ulcer pain diminishes, the four-times-a-day antacid regime would be started.

The amount of antacid that you take each time will depend upon the specific antacid that you are using. As I stated before, antacid preparations have different capacities to buffer your stomach acid.[11] The weaker antacids would require a dosage of three to four teaspoons instead of the half a teaspoon dosage for a stronger or more potent antacid. This will account for the difference noted among antacid users. It is very important to remember to ask your doctor or pharmacist about the strength of your antacid and the proper amount to be taken.

Side Effects of Antacids

Antacids are the mainstay in the treatment of peptic ulcer disease. They are usually safe and effective when utilized properly. However, there are some side effects that can occur with antacid therapy. One of the most frequently observed consequences of antacid usage is the change in bowel function and regularity. Commonly the magnesium containing antacids will exert a mild laxative action while the aluminum-based antacids will have a constipating effect. Therefore, many individuals have found it best to alternate these different types of antacids and maintain their normal bowel habits. The salt or sodium content of various antacids differs greatly. This is a very important consideration in those individuals who require antacid therapy but need to restrict their sodium intake because of associated diseases such as high blood pressure or heart failure. Your pharmacist or doctor can help to select the proper antacid for use in these special circumstances.

Calcium carbonate is the strongest antacid in regard to its acid-neutralizing capabilities. However, after buffering the existing acid within the stomach, the calcium component stimulates the stomach to produce more acid.[12] This stimulatory effect usually occurs one hour after the ingestion of the antacid. This would explain the commonly observed need for those people to repeatedly take more antacid. For this reason, many ulcer specialists do not recommend the regular usage of calcium carbonate antacids. Remember to check the active ingredient in your favorite antacid preparation.

There is another reason to avoid the prolonged high-dose usage of calcium-containing antacids. An increase in the blood calcium level could result. This side effect would develop as more and more calcium is absorbed through the stomach lining. If this did occur, kidney stones would likely develop. It is possible that the calcium could settle out in other body organs and cause tissue injury. These reasons, coupled with the previously described "rebound effect" on gastric or stomach acid production, make calcium containing antacids less favorably viewed by many digestive disease experts.

The aluminum-containing antacids may—I repeat may—cause softening of the bones with prolonged usage.[13] This softening of the bones would result from the binding of the phosphorus, contained within our foods, by the antacids and decrease the amount of phosphorus that could be absorbed by the digestive process. Phosphorus is an important element in the supporting structure or framework of our bones. A decrease in the amount present in our bones would make them softer and could predispose them to fracture more easily.

Baking soda or sodium carbonate has been used as an antacid in the past by many individuals. This practice should be strongly discouraged because of serious potential side effects. It is true that baking soda is a very effective antacid. However, it produces secondary stomach acid secretion, similar to the calcium-containing antacids, which means it has a short-term antacid effect. Its salt content makes this a potentially dangerous antacid for use by those people who cannot tolerate the extra sodium. The prolonged usage of sodium carbonate could result in acid-base imbalance within the blood and adversely affect the functions of the kidneys. Therefore, the regular usage of baking soda as an antacid is strongly discouraged, for you may "cook your own cake" with it.

An important consideration to remember is that your antacid may interact with other medications that you may be taking. The antacid may alter the rate of uptake from the GI tract and cause important fluctuations in the blood level of that drug. These changes in the blood level could cause side effects from that medication or prevent the drug from doing its job. Therefore, antacids should not be taken randomly or without good medical reasons. This medication, which antacids are, should be taken regularly only at the advice of a physician. It is sound advice to have your questions about antacids or their use answered by a pharmacist or doctor.

Your physician will probably elect to use another medication in addition to your antacid therapy in the treatment of a peptic ulcer. In the past this medication would have been an anticholinergic preparation.[14] This type of drug decreases the secretion of stomach acid but has undesirable side effects. Dryness of the mouth and eyes, blurring of vision, headaches, and difficulty with urination were commonly observed in individuals taking this type of medication. Though still used today in the treatment of peptic ulcer disease, anticholinergic drugs have been mainly replaced by the newer "miracle" ulcer drugs.

Tagament, or Cimetidine, was the first new drug that was released in the United States to be used in the therapy of duodenal ulcer disease. This medication, which is made by the Smith, Kline, and French Drug Company, was released seven years ago with great publicity. This drug had a very impressive record in European trials in the treatment of peptic ulcer disease. To this date, both duodenal ulcer patients and physicians alike have been tremendously satisfied with the use of Tagament in the United States. Very recently the Food and Drug Administration approved the use of Tagament, or Cimetidine, for the treatment of gastric ulcerations. All of us dealing with peptic ulcer disease welcome this announcement with open arms. Indeed, this miracle ulcer drug has lived up to its billing.

This new drug works by decreasing the stomach acid production to a minute quantity.[15] One tablet taken orally will result in virtually no stomach acid being produced for four hours. This medication is usually given to patients with active ulcer disease for a four-to six-week time period. One tablet is taken with each meal and at bedtime.

Many happy patients will attest to the effectiveness of Tagament in the treatment of ulcer disease. Most wish that the drug had been discovered years before. The one complaint of most takers of the drug has been its price. On the average, a four- to six-week prescription of Tagament will cost between \$26 and \$34. To many, this cost has been worth the freedom from their ulcer pain and their return to good health.

Today in the United States, Tagament is the number one selling pharmaceutical drug in the country.[16] This fact is causing great concern among digestive disease experts. Unfortunately this probably means that the drug is not being utilized properly and in accord with F.D.A. indications. The indiscriminate taking of Tagament in high doses is to be strongly discouraged.[17] This statement is made because there is a known 5 percent incidence of adverse reactions to this medication.[18] Though the majority of these reactions are minor and usually reversible, there is a concern about less frequent but more serious effects. The long-term effects of high dose Tagament therapy on important body organs such as the bone marrow and stomach remain to be definitely determined.

Tagament is approved for use in a reduced-dose form and in a one-time-a-day formulation. This type of therapy with Tagament has been shown to be effective in reducing the incidence of recurrence of duodenal ulcerations. This fact may prove to be one of the drug's strongest attributes. This form of therapy is usually begun after the completion of the regular four to six weeks of one tablet four times a day. This is not the long-term therapy that digestive disease experts are concerned about. It is the continuation of one tablet four times a day in the regular strength that these physicians strongly discourage. If you have any questions regarding the frequency or the dosage of Tagament, or Cimetidine, that you should be taking, consult your doctor.

About two years ago Carafate, or Sucralfate, was released by the Food and Drug Administration for the treatment of duodenal ulcer disease. This drug is made by Marion Laboratories, Inc. This medication had been used in Japan for many years with a proven efficacy record and a history of minor side effects occurring rarely. This drug works by a different mechanism than does Tagament. Carafate does not affect stomach acid production but rather forms a protective covering for the ulcer. This antiacid barrier enables the ulceration to heal.

Carafate is prescribed in a dosage of one tablet four times a day, one hour before meals and on an empty stomach at bedtime. It is usually taken for four to six weeks. To date, the experience with Sucralfate has shown it be effective in the healing of duodenal ulcers and to be a safe drug with few adverse reactions. However, because of the prior existence of Tagament, Carafate has not become as widely used.

There will soon be a "second cousin" of Tagament, or Cimetidine, on the market to be used in the therapy of peptic ulcer disease.[19] This drug is called ranitidine and will be made by Glaxo Pharmaceuticals. This new ulcer drug will work in a way similar to Tagament but will be stronger and need to be taken less frequently. It is expected that the F.D.A. will shortly give its approval to this drug. Where it will fit into the treatment scheme of peptic ulcer disease will be determined in the future.

All of the newer ulcer therapy medications have been a welcomed advance in the treatment of peptic ulcer disease. They have not reduced the need for ulcer operations as was frequently discussed during their clinical trials or early years of usage. Surgery is still required for the effective control of ulcer disease in certain individuals. When should an ulcer operation be performed? Surgery is still required for the complications of peptic ulcer disease. However, before proceeding with a discussion of the role of surgery in the treatment of ulcer disease, I would now like to mention the complications of this illness.

Complications of Peptic Ulcer Disease

Importantly, a complication of peptic ulcer disease occurs in about 5 to 10 percent of individuals.[20] The complications include bleeding, scarring with blockage of the intestinal tract, and perforation of the GI tract. Bleeding ulcerations result when the ulcer erodes into a vessel in the lining of the stomach or duodenum. Blockage or obstruction results from the scarring associated with the healing of some duodenal ulcerations. Perforation of the intestinal tract occurs when the ulcer erodes completely through the wall of either the stomach or duodenum. No one can predict which individual with ulcer disease will experience a complication. What are the indications that some one has a complication of peptic ulcer disease? What are their symptoms?

The most common complication of duodenal ulcer disease and the one associated with the greatest need for hospitalization is bleeding. The bleeding rate may be slow and stop spontaneously. In other patients, the rate of bleeding will be profuse and constant. It is these individuals that will go into shock and possibly die unless vigorous medical treatment is given. Persons with a slow bleeding ulceration will typically notice the presence of a dark tarry black stool. This type of stool will also be more difficult to clean with the bathroom tissue. The color and the physical characteristics of this type of stool result from the blood, within the bowel or intestinal tract, being acted upon by bacteria. This melanotic stool, as it is known in the medical profession, should always be looked for by ulcer disease patients. In addition, individuals with slow bleeding ulcerations may notice a sick feeling to their stomach and have vomiting. The contents of the vomitus will usually look like coffee grounds and contain a small amount of bright red blood within it. The coffee ground appearance is due to the old blood within the stomach being acted upon by the stomach acid. Any ulcer patient who notices any of these signs should contact a physician or go to an emergency room immediately. A rapidly bleeding ulceration of the stomach or duodenum will cause a different group of signs and symptoms. People will notice the passage of bright red blood per rectum or the movement of a maroon-colored stool. They will have an increased frequency of bowel movements during the acute bleeding episode because the blood within the intestinal tract causes it to have more contractions. They may vomit bright red blood with a large clot within it. If the bleeding rate continues to be fast and nonstopping, some will notice a lightheadedness with standing. A few may actually pass out. Not uncommonly, the individual will go to the bathroom and be found passed out on the floor. Needless to say, these symptoms require immediate medical attention.

The most dramatic complication of peptic ulcer disease is a perforation of the intestinal tract. This results in the establishment of a connection between the GI tract and the abdominal cavity. The intestinal contents, acid and digestive enzymes, irritate the lining of the abdominal cavity. This lining is known as the peritoneum and the inflammation is called peritonitis. This situation causes severe unremitting abdominal pain and can result in shock and death. The pain associated with peritonitis is different than the person's typical ulcer pain. This pain is usually increased with walking or any movement that will jar the abdominal contents. This complication of peptic ulcer disease is a medical emergency that requires prompt attention. Surgery is required to close the opening in the GI tract wall and to drain the inflamed peritoneal lining. Fortunately, most individuals make a successful recovery after surgery. Unfortunately, this complication was not recognized in my father and he died as a result of it. Therefore, my main reason to write this book becomes evident.

The last complication of peptic ulcer disease is obstruction of the stomach or duodenum. This is seen after the active ulcer has healed. Ulcer patients will notice a sensation of fullness after eating and may have associated nausea and vomiting. They decrease the amount of food that they eat and lose weight. The weight lost is a result of both the decreased caloric intake and the inability of the food to pass into the intestines and be properly taken up. Any ulcer patient noticing these symptoms should contact a physician. Surgery may be indicated to correct the blockage and restore that person to a normal state of health.

Surgery for Peptic Ulcers

As you have learned, surgery is required for a perforated ulcer and may be necessary for an uncontrolled bleeding ulceration. Surgery will probably be needed to correct the obstruction that results from the healing of some peptic ulcers. The timing of an elective surgical procedure for uncomplicated peptic ulcer disease remains a difficult decision for patient and physician. Some people will not have relief of their ulcer pain despite faithful adherence to an appropriate ulcer treatment program. Surgery will be considered in these "intractable pain" cases.[21] The timing of this elective surgery will be dependent upon the amount of time these individuals have lost from dutiful employment and their acceptance of "the ulcer way of life." Many sufferers of peptic ulcer disease can finally not accept the continuous pain and the alterations in their life style. An ulcer operation would be an appropriate consideration for those individuals.

The majority of ulcer patients who have an ulcer operation are satisfied with the results of their surgery. However, a small percentage will not be freed of their symptoms and may develop new stomach pains as a consequence of the surgery. This new pain results when the lining of the stomach becomes inflamed by the action of the bile. It is common after ulcer operations to have an abnormal amount of bile present in the stomach. This condition is known as bile gastritis. When it occurs, bile gastritis may produce symptoms that are worse than the original ulcer pain. Other symptoms may occur after an ulcer operation. Some people will notice a persistent and bothersome diarrhea that occurs regularly after eating. Other individuals will experience a low blood sugar level and feel faint and lightheaded after eating. These symptoms, which are known to affect certain individuals after ulcer surgery, are referred to in medical talk as the dumping syndrome. Finally, somewhere between 1 and 5 percent of people will develop a recurrence of their ulcerations sometime in the postoperative period.[23]

Therefore, all elective ulcer surgery should be decided on the basis of "hard data," with open discussions between the patient and doctor. All of the possible complications and sequela of ulcer surgery should be adequately explained to the patients. In this way, that individual can make a decision knowing all the facts.

Summary

Peptic ulcer disease is a common ailment that affects millions of Americans. This disease may have a great economic impact on those people. It will alter their life styles to varying degrees. The complications of ulcer disease may be life-threatening. Antacids remain a mainstay in the treatment of ulcer disease. The newer ulcer drugs have been a welcomed advance. Surgery is required to treat some of the complications of ulcer disease and to cure others with the disease. If you are one of the unfortunate individuals with peptic ulcer disease, I am hopeful the contents of this chapter will improve your understanding of the disease and maybe improve your life style.

chapter three

Heartburn

Heartburn, the sensation of warmth or a warm fluid moving upward beneath the breastbone, is one digestive symptom most of us have experienced at some time.[1] People experiencing heartburn on a regular basis describe their symptoms as a "fire bellowing upward from my stomach" or state, "I am on fire underneath my breastbone."[2,3] Approximately 10 percent of Americans experience heartburn on a regular basis.[4] The majority of us have suffered with it only occasionally.

Function of the Esophagus

Why does heartburn occur? In order to understand this digestive symptom, we will first review the location and function of the food tube or esophagus. The gullet, the food tube, or esophagus are all names of the organ that carries the food from the mouth to the stomach. This organ, lying behind the chest cavity, connects the mouth to the abdominal cavity. The diaphragm, the large sheet muscle that separates these two body cavities and is responsible for respirations, has an opening through which the food tube, or esophagus, passes. The esophagus's only function is for the transportation of food. No digestive process occurs within this organ. The rhythmic contractions of the gullet propel the food downward from the mouth to the stomach.

Normally, once the food has entered the stomach, the reentrance of the food, digestive enzymes, or stomach acid into the esophagus is prevented by the muscle tone at the junction of the esophagus and stomach. This muscle tone of the lower food tube is known as the lower esophageal sphincter or L.E.S. It acts as a valve to prevent the reflux of stomach contents into the esophagus.

This valve action is generated by a zone of high pressure created across the end of the esophagus by this sphincter.[5,6,7]

Certain factors influence this sphincter to decrease the pressure that is normally generated to a low enough level that stomach contents can reflux, or move upward, into the esophagus. The gastric juices, with their hydrochloric acid content, irritate and inflame the lining of the esophagus, resulting in the sensation of heartburn.

Factors That Contribute to Heartburn

Which social habits or factors can predispose to heartburn? The foods we eat have an important effect on the function of the lower esophageal sphincter. Fatty foods, chocolates, caffeine-containing beverages and after-dinner mints reduce the ability of the esophagus to prevent reflux. Heartburn may result after eating these foods. Clearly, the individual who recognized the value of the after-dinner belch, knew the influence of mints on the function of the lower esophagus. Both smoking and alcoholic consumption can result in the

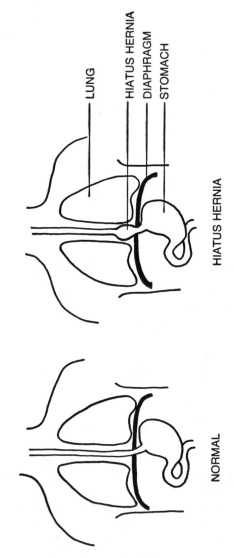

LUNG

HIATUS HERNIA

DIAPHRAGM

STOMACH

HIATUS HERNIA

NORMAL

ILLUSTRATION 3. Hiatus Hernia.

reflux of gastric contents into the esophagus. In addition, both of these social habits increase the amount of acid secreted by the stomach. Therefore, in patients experiencing heartburn regularly, drinking and alcoholic consumption tend to prolong and increase the severity of their heartburn. Former smokers are frequently pleasantly surprised with the disappearance of their frequently occurring heartburn symptom. Therefore, all of us who experience heartburn regularly must closely evaluate our social habits and watch specific types of foods that we eat. Medications have varying effects on the esophagus and its ability to prevent reflux. Millions of Americans are on various muscle relaxant drugs or antianxiety medications. The majority of these drugs decrease the ability of the esophagus to prevent reflux. Certain patients taking this type of medication will notice heartburn as a consequence of that drug's usage. Physicians prescribe anticholinergic drugs for many individuals with various GI complaints. This type of drug, commonly known as an antispasmodic drug, is used to decrease bowel motility and intestinal secretions. All of these drugs predispose the taker to reflux of gastric contents into the esophagus. Commonly, individuals taking this type of medication on a regular basis will develop troublesome heartburn. The newer cardiac drugs, or antiangina calcium-blockers, will also lower the esophageal pressure and enable esophageal reflux. If you are one of the unfortunate individuals who requires the regular usage of any of these medications, consult your physician if persistent heartburn results.

An individual's weight is another important consideration in examining the causes of persistent heartburn. Excess body weight or obesity, especially in the form of a "potbelly," causes increased pressure to be transmitted to the stomach through the abdominal wall. This extra pressure is especially important when the individual is lying down. The pressure can force gastric contents up into the esophagus by overcoming the pressure generated at the junction of the esophagus and stomach. It is important that all individuals suffering from persistent heartburn achieve an ideal body weight in an attempt to eliminate this factor as a cause of their heartburn. Certain individuals with persistent heartburn will notice that changes in body position will increase the severity of this symptom. These individuals notice increased heartburn while bending over to tie their shoes or bending over to pick something off the floor. Usually, these same individuals will notice increased severity of their heartburn with lying down. Sleeping flat in a bed is often difficult for these unfortunate people. The symptoms of heartburn are increased because of the dependent position of the esophagus in relationship to the stomach in these various positions. More simply stated, it is easier for the gastric juices to flow downhill into the esophagus.

The majority of pregnant women have experienced the symptom of heartburn. Heartburn occurs so commonly during pregnancy because of the effects of the female hormones on the esophagus. These hormonal effects predispose individuals to the reflux of gastric secretions into the esophagus with its attendant heartburn symptom. The upward displacement of the stomach by the enlarging pregnant uterus, or womb, also predisposes these women to increased esophageal reflux. Importantly, most women experiencing heartburn symptoms during their pregnancy will notice relief of their heartburn with the birth of their baby.

The Hiatus Hernia

What is a hiatus hernia and what is its relationship to heartburn and esophageal reflux? A hiatus hernia exists when the upper portion of the stomach slips upward, through the opening in the diaphragm, and rests in the chest cavity instead of the belly cavity. The slippage of the stomach into the chest cavity may occur intermittently or be a permanent feature of one's anatomy. What causes the opening in the diaphragm to weaken or widen and allow this upward movement is not fully understood. Certainly some individuals are born with a weakened opening that will predispose them to the development of a hiatus hernia over the years. There is a common misconception that a hiatus hernia, like inguinal or groin hernias, result from heavy lifting. There is no scientific data that would substantiate this belief. It is recognized that a severe traumatic blow to the abdomen can result in the development of a hiatus hernia.

The likelihood of having a hiatus hernia increases with age.[8] Approximately 20 to 30 percent of Americans below the age of forty will have a hiatus hernia, compared with the 50 to 60 percent of individuals over seventy years of age. It would appear that the aging process affects the diaphragm as it affects our other muscles. As we lose our muscle tone in our arms and legs, the muscle tone of the diaphragm might decrease to explain the observed increased incidence of hiatus hernia in older individuals.

Does a hiatus hernia have any functional significance or is it just a variant of our normal anatomy? Or stated in another way, does the presence of the stomach in the chest cavity predispose an individual to the development of esophageal reflux and heartburn? Most individuals are of the misconception that they need a hiatus hernia to have esophageal reflux or heartburn. The presence of the upper portion of the stomach within the chest cavity does not affect the normal functioning of the lower esophagus. Therefore, a hiatus hernia is only a variant of our normal anatomy. The presence of a hiatus hernia does not necessarily predispose to esophageal reflux and heartburn. A hiatus hernia and an abnormal functioning lower esophagus are required in order to have esophageal reflux.

It is most important that we do not equate the presence of a hiatus hernia with esophageal reflux and heartburn. These terms are not synonymous. This is one of the most common misconceptions that the American public has regarding their health. In the past, all sufferers of esophageal reflux were felt to have a hiatus hernia. Today we know that people with a hiatus hernia do not suffer from esophageal reflux and heartburn unless their lower esophagus does not function properly. It is the normal functioning of the esophageal sphincter that prevents reflux, even in those individuals with the anatomical variant known as a hiatus hernia.

Preventing Esophageal Reflux and Heartburn

What can be done to prevent esophageal reflux and heartburn from occurring? Sufferers of persistent heartburn must make certain changes in their daily life styles to decrease the frequency and severity of this symptom. A change in the daily diet is an important first step. A low-fat, high-protein diet is recommended because of its positive effect on the functioning of the lower esophagus. This diet should include avoidance of greasy foods, all chocolate-containing foods, and all mint treats. A strict adherence to such a diet should also allow for a slow weight loss that will be helpful to overweight individuals. At first it will be difficult to refuse those delicious chocolate sweets and the after-dinner mints. Most sufferers of persistent heartburn accept these dietary adjustments when they notice the improvement that results.

Importantly no food should be eaten for about one hour before retiring to bed for the night. The reasoning is that the maximum amount of acid produced by the stomach occurs one hour after eating. Therefore, if a large bedtime snack is consumed shortly before retiring, the high acid content of the stomach would increase the severity of the heartburn. Many individuals who formerly experienced severe heartburn symptoms during the night have benefited greatly from this dietary restriction.

Besides the aforementioned dietary changes, a change in our social habits will have a great influence on the frequency and the severity of heartburn that we experience. By decreasing the consumption of caffeine-containing foods, we will remove one factor that can predispose to heartburn. Smoking should be decreased or stopped completely in an attempt to eliminate another factor that could increase the frequency and severity of heartburn.

Many important considerations for the prevention of esophageal reflux or heartburn have just been outlined. These recommendations must be followed in order to achieve a successful resolution of heartburn problems. What else can be done to help us eliminate the heartache of heartburn? Antacids remain an important factor in the treatment of heartburn and esophageal reflux. Antacids do two things to help heartburn. First they neutralize or decrease the acid in the stomach. Therefore, if the reflux of gastric juices into the esophagus occurs, the gastric juices are less acidic and less irritating to the lining of the esophagus. Secondly, antacids act on the lower esophagus to increase the pressure between the stomach and esophagus and to prevent esophageal reflux and heartburn.

The choice and the usage of antacids has been previously discussed in Chapter 2.

Some individuals experiencing severe heartburn at night benefit by the placement of four to six inch blocks under the head of their bed frame. This creates a situation that prevents reflux because the fluid does not run uphill. This simple maneuver has given many sufferers of nighttime reflux dramatic relief. Many of my patients have been concerned about the potential problem that this would cause in the accomplishment of nighttime pleasantries. I assure you, elevating the head of the bed four to six inches does not produce a ski-slope effect. Some individuals have tried to achieve this same affect by sleeping with two to three pillows. Usually this does not achieve the same degree of success as putting the blocks under the head of the bedpost.

Reflux Esophagitis
and Its Treatment

Are there complications of persistent reflux of gastric contents into the esophagus? Does persistent heartburn indicate there is something seriously wrong with our esophagus? The continuous irritation of the lining of the esophagus by the stomach juices and acid can result in a condition known as reflux esophagitis.[9,10] Inflammation of the lining of the esophagus does not occur in all individuals with heartburn. Only in those individuals with severe and persistent esophageal reflux will reflux esophagitis occur. It is important to prevent inflammation of the lining of the esophagus. Reflux esophagitis can be associated with complications; however, intermittent esophageal reflux will not do us any significant harm.

It is difficult to state the exact percentage of individuals with esophageal reflux that will develop reflux esophagitis. Surely, the treatment of esophageal reflux is simple enough to prevent the possibility of resulting peptic esophagitis. Individuals with reflux esophagitis will notice the presence of heartburn and intermittent difficulty with swallowing foods and liquids. This difficulty in swallowing results from the spasm, or altered motility, of the esophagus as a consequence of the inflammation. As the inflammation worsens, individuals may notice that certain foods will burn as they pass downward. Usually these are acid-containing foods such as citrus fruits and their juices, tomatoes, and tomato juices and hot liquids. Anyone experiencing heartburn plus difficulty swallowing or the sensation of the food burning as it passes from the mouth to the stomach should consult a physician. These symptoms indicate that the inflammation within the esophagus is severe.

The treatment of reflux esophagitis will involve the dietary suggestions and restrictions as outlined for heartburn and simple esophageal reflux. Also, antacids will be given to help reduce the inflammation within the esophagus. In addition, your physician may elect to add various medications that will help to either reduce the amount of reflux into the esophagus or help reduce the acidity of the gastric contents. Gaviscon, a product of Marion Laboratories, Inc., is an over-the-counter antiesophageal reflux drug. This medication reacts with the acid within the stomach to form a protective antireflux foam barrier in the top portion of the stomach. This product is not a potent antacid and should be used in conjunction with antacid treatment. Tagamet has been widely used in the treatment of reflux esophagitis. It is most commonly prescribed in a manner similar to its use in the treatment of active peptic ulcer disease.

Esophageal Stricture and Its Treatment

The majority of individuals will respond to the treatment program for their reflux esophagitis. Unfortunately, certain individuals live with their reflux esophagitis too long and complications develop. Approximately 5 to 10 percent of individuals with persistent and severe reflux esophagitis will develop a complication from the persistent inflammation of the lining of the gullet. A narrowing of the esophagus can result from this chronic inflammation. This narrowing is called an esophageal stricture. Most of these strictures are long, but sometimes are very narrow and resemble an inflammatory ring within the esophagus. This esophageal ring is known as a Schatzki's ring. Esophageal strictures are the most common complication of severe reflux esophagitis. People with these strictures will notice persistent difficulties in swallowing solid foods such as meats. People with esophageal strictures state, "Doc, the food sticks here," pointing to the lower end of the breastbone. This is the area where they experience the sensation of their food stopping and not passing into the stomach. Some of these individuals will have to regurgitate this undigested food to obtain relief. Others will change their eating habits to include a lot of fluids in an attempt to wash down the slowly advancing solid foods. Eventually, most people with a marked narrowing of their esophagus will eliminate meats totally from their diet. Some will be fortunate enough to be able to continue to eat broiled chicken or ground meat without problems.

Rarely people with esophageal strictures will have a piece of meat lodge in their esophagus that will not advance. This is associated with severe pain and discomfort beneath the breastbone. This situation requires immediate medical attention. In some individuals the administration of a muscle relaxant will allow for the passage of the lodged meat. In the majority, however, the impacted or lodged meat particle must be removed with flexible instruments known as endoscopes. These important diagnostic and treatment tools were discussed in Chapter 2.

Some individuals with an esophageal stricture will not totally pass the ingested food into their stomach. Then, with recumbancy, portions of this nondigested food may move upward from the esophagus and into the air tubes while sleeping. The unknowing aspiration of food may lead to a pneumonia or scarring of the lungs.

Esophageal strictures can be successfully treated in the majority of cases by medical management. This treatment is known as esophageal dilatation or bougienage. Rubber mercury-filled tubes, or dilators, are passed through the mouth into the esophagus. Before esophageal dilatation occurs, the patient is given a liquid novacaine solution to numb the back of the throat. Esophageal dilators of increasing size are passed through into the esophagus to stretch the esophageal narrowing. This procedure must be done slowly and usually over many sittings so that the stretching of the stricture is done slowly and the esophagus is not torn. Despite the seemingly awful description of esophageal dilatation, the majority of patients with esophageal strictures welcome the relief obtained by the procedure. Some of the most grateful patients are those who are now able to enjoy a steak dinner instead of a ground meat special. Unfortunately, certain individuals will not respond to esophageal dilatation and will require surgery to dilate their esophageal narrowing.

A rare complication of reflux esophagitis is a peptic ulceration occurring in the esophagus. People with a peptic ulcer of the esophagus will experience severe continuous pain beneath their breastbone. The intensity and severity of the pain may make the individual and doctors feel that the pain is due to a heart attack. Only after an X-ray of the esophagus is done will the correct diagnosis be known. These ulcers of the esophagus will usually respond to a treatment program similar to that for peptic ulcer disease of the duodenum.

Reflux esophagitis can result in bleeding from the inflamed lining of the esophagus. The bleeding may be slow or brisk. Therefore, either black tarry bowel movements or vomiting of blood could result from bleeding from the lining of the esophagus. Any patient with heartburn noticing these signs should consult a physician immediately. It is important to note that most sufferers of reflux esophagitis who experience bleeding from their upper gastrointestinal tract will have a source of the bleeding found to be other than their esophagus. That is, some will be found to have a bleeding duodenal ulcer or bleeding from the lining of the stomach.

Another recognized complication of reflux esophagitis is a condition known as a Barrett's esophagus. Dr. Barrett was the English surgeon who first recognized this complication. In this condition the lining of the esophagus changes to resemble the lining of the stomach. This change of tissue appearance is called a metaplastic change. This change is believed to occur as a result of the continuous inflammation of the lining of the esophagus. The importance of this change is that somewhere between 8 to 20 percent of people having a Barrett's esophagus will be found to have a malignant tumor of the esophagus.[11,12] This is the most important reason to prevent severe and prolonged reflux esophagitis. No one is able to predict which individuals with severe reflux esophagitis will develop a Barrett's esophagus.

Summary

Heartburn is a symptom of esophageal reflux. The abnormal functioning of the lower esophagus predisposes to reflux. A hiatus hernia is a variant of our normal anatomy and does not cause esophageal reflux unless there is an associated abnormal functioning of the lower esophagus. Persistent esophageal reflux may damage the lining of the esophagus, resulting in an esophagitis. Severe reflux esophagitis may be associated with important complications. Our diet and social habits are important factors associated with esophageal reflux, and therefore reflux esophagitis. Anyone experiencing persistent problems in swallowing food should consult a physician immediately.

chapter four
Intestinal Gas

Complaints attributable to excessive intestinal gas are one of the most frequently mentioned health symptoms. These complaints will vary from bloating to belching and the need to express gas per rectum.
It is interesting to notice the difference in various societies' and cultures' acceptance of belching and flatulence, the process of passing gas per rectum. The Chinese have long accepted the after-dinner belch as an expression of satisfaction with the meal. The Romans accepted flatulence as acceptable etiquette. But today's society does not accept the view "do as the Romans do."
Most individuals have the misconception that their gas problems are a result of their stomach not working properly. "Extra gas on the stomach" is a phrase commonly used by individuals to explain their special problem while out in

public. The source of the problem in most cases is not the stomach, but rather the intestines.

Causes of Intestinal Gas

Normally the sugars taken in with our diets are absorbed or processed for use within the small intestine. If a large volume of sugar is ingested, the capacity of the small intestine to take up all the sugars may be exceeded. The sugars that remain in the intestine are fermented by the bacteria within the large bowel. This fermentation process results in the production of intestinal gas. The majority of the gas made is hydrogen, with a small amount of carbon dioxide resulting. In addition to the gases being formed, certain acids are produced. The importance of these acids will be explained later in this chapter.

The excessive sugar can be ingested in a variety of forms. Most of us have experienced flatulence the morning after a beer party or after having drunk a large quantity of wine at a social occasion. The sugars in those socially acceptable beverages were responsible for this. A variety of fruits and vegetables contain sugars that may not be totally taken up by the small intestine. These foods are noteworthy causes of flatulence. This association has best been described by the slang expression: "Beans, beans, the musical fruit. The more you eat, the more you toot." But it is no laughing matter for those less fortunate individuals.

Treatment for Excessive Intestinal Gas

It becomes evident that our diet plays an important part in the cause of flatulence. If you suffer with this social problem, remember to check the types of foods that you are eating. You will probably be amazed at the amount of sugar that you are consuming. Do not forget the artificial sweeteners in all the diet sodas or the regular or sugarless gums that you chew. Take the time to adequately check your diet. This time will be well spent if you can prevent future episodes of social embarrassment.

A common cause of flatulence is the inability of certain people to tolerate the sugar in milk or milk products such as cheese or ice cream. The sugar is called lactose and the condition is known as lactose intolerance. Those individuals cannot absorb that sugar in their intestine. The flatulence results from the fermentation of the nonabsorbed milk sugar. This condition, lactose intolerance, will be reviewed in detail in Chapter 8, for it is a frequent cause of many GI complaints besides flatulence.

Rarely does an intestinal gas problem result from a specific disease of the small intestine. However, people known to have intestinal diseases will experience flatulence after the ingestion of certain foods containing sugar. The disease causes the small intestine not to handle the sugars properly. Therefore, people with Crohn's disease of the small intestine will have to make dietary adjustments. This disease will be discussed fully in Chapter 13.

Since most people with flatulence or bloating will have their problem as a result of the body handling the excess sugar they eat, a change is required in their diet. Most will notice an improvement in their symptoms by adhering to a low-carbohydrate or low-sugar diet. Those intolerant of milk will improve when milk is removed from their diet. Remember to take the time to review your dietary intake completely.

Treatment of Bloating and Abdominal Pain

Can excess intestinal gas result in bloating and abdominal pain? Indeed, it will commonly result in these symptoms. This combination, "too much gas, bloating, and crampy abdominal pain," is one of the most frequent reasons why people consult a digestive disease specialist.[1] It has been estimated that one third to one half of patients' visits to the previously mentioned physicians will be because of these complaints. The bloating is usually described as occurring one to two hours after eating. This sensation of bloating is frequently associated with crampy abdominal pains and flatulence. The excess gas causes the bowel to distend and produces the discomfort. A majority of these individuals will notice an improvement of their symptoms with the passage of gas per rectum or flatus. Relief will also be noticed after having a bowel movement. An X-ray of the abdomen, taken in the same way as a simple chest X-ray, would demonstrate a large amount of gas within the large intestine. Other invididuals will not have a large amount of gas within the large bowel as determined by the abdominal X-ray. In these persons the extra gas would produce abnormal contractions or spasms of the intestine. Their crampy pains and bloating would result from these spasms. Most of these individuals would not experience relief with the passage of flatus or having a bowel movement.[2]

The treatment of those people with gas-related abdominal pain and bloating or abdominal distension is twofold. First their diet is changed to lower the amount of sugar that they ingest. Secondly drugs that are designed to reduce the severity of their bowel spasms would be prescribed. It is impossible to predict which individuals will respond to those medications. Some will be helped, while others will continue to have gas-related complaints.

What is the relationship of belching to intestinal gas? Most people who experience frequent episodes of belching do so not because of a problem with excessive intestinal gas, but rather, because they actually swallow air before each belch. This air swallowing is done unconsciously in the majority of cases. Therefore, they are expressing the air that they swallowed immediately before the belch, or eructation, as it is known medically. Many, but not all, air swallowers suffer from chronic anxiety. This air swallowing, or aerophagia, as it is known, occurs as a consequence of the tension they feel. These individuals would benefit most from psychological consultation. Medicines or dietary changes will not help the majority of these people.[3]

Rarely air swallowing will be the cause of a person's flatulence.[4] This requires the ingestion of an enormous amount of air. The volume of air is such that all of it is not absorbed by the intestine. The resulting air that reaches the large bowel may be expressed as flatus. This individual would almost certainly benefit from counseling.

There are certain over-the-counter preparations that are sold to assist the person who has an excess intestinal gas problem. These will contain various charcoal mixtures or combinations of low-dose digestive enzymes. Many will contain simthicone, the antigas compound. The response to these preparations is not very predictable. If you are fortunate enough to find one that seems to help, I would recommend that you use it as directed. My experience has shown that dietary changes and anxiety control are important first steps in the control of excess intestinal gas.

No chapter on intestinal gas would be complete without mentioning the "blue-flamer" fad of the late 1950s and early 1960s. This craze reflected a change in approach to entertainment by some members of our society. This fad consisted of lighting flatus with a match. It was popularly practiced in locker rooms, summer camps, and military training facilities. The aim was to produce a "blue-flamer." Those capable of such a feat were held in high regard, but many suffered anal irritation secondary only to heatburn.

Methane gas, a gas produced within the large bowel, was responsible for the heralded flame. The ability to produce methane gas is inherited as a familial characteristic. The hope of many small boys during this time was to find out that their older brother was a "blue-flamer." It is hoped that this form of entertainment has been replaced by video games or traditional sporting contests. In theory it was possible for a colonic explosion to occur in certain individuals. This form of social diversion should be strongly discouraged.

Summary

Intestinal gas is a frequent cause of social embarrassment to many individuals. In addition, it is a common reason why many will have bloating and abdominal pain. Remember the importance of the sugar content of your diet. If dietary changes or over-the-counter preparations do not result in relief of your symptoms, consult a physician. It is hoped that the information contained within this chapter will allow the readers to be able to prevent future social embarrassment.

chapter five
Bowel Irregularity

Americans, more than any other citizen group, are preoccupied with the necessity for bowel regularity. Changes in bowel habits greatly influence productivity in our daily lives. Bowel irregularity may have a tremendous impact on one's personality and our social interactions. All of us can remember the moodiness and shortness of temper associated with a bout of constipation. When diarrhea occurs, our interest and desire to perform our job decreases.

We must first try to define bowel regularity. What is a normal bowel habit for an average adult American? This is truly one of the most difficult questions relating to our health to answer with certainty and valid scientific data. Many well-designed studies have been completed in an attempt to try to answer this question. The results of these studies have shown the average number of bowel movements for an adult American to be three to four times a week.[1]

Therefore, the absence of a daily bowel movement is not abnormal for many Americans. These studies also demonstrated that our diet plays an important role in determining frequency of our bowel habits. Individuals consuming a high-fiber diet have, on the average, more frequent bowel movements and bulkier stools than individuals eating a low-fiber diet.

An important consideration for us to remember is that each of us have a bowel habit or frequency that is right for us. Some may have a bowel movement once every ten to fourteen days without experiencing symptoms of discomfort or fullness. Others may have one to three bowel movements daily for the majority of their life. The important factor is that the frequency of the bowel movements is regular and not associated with any abnormal complaints.

All of us will notice variations in our regular bowel habits. These variations are the loose stools associated with a viral illness, the increased stool frequency when nervous or under emotional stress, variations in our stool size and frequency with changes in our diet, and occasional episodes of constipation associated with periods of prolonged inactivity or decreased fluid intake. All of these changes in our bowel habits are temporary and are usually associated with a quick return to our normal routine.

Many Americans are not so fortunate and suffer with regular constipation. The magnitude and the impact of this bowel irregularity is reflected by the sales of over $250 million worth of over-the-counter laxatives yearly.[2] Some regular users of laxatives have a lifelong problem with constipation, while others reflect the need for laxative usage beginning in the middle of their life. Is there any reason for this difference?

Causes of Constipation

Some digestive disease experts feel that people with a lifelong problem with constipation have this bowel irregularity as a result of their toilet training procedure. Usually, but not invariably, many of these individuals had strict toilet training with a great deal of attention being given to the accidental stool soilings. As a child, they develop the habit of stool holding to prevent future accidents and to reduce the displeasure of their parents. Gradually the appreciation of rectal fullness, the normal stimulant for a bowel movement, is reduced with the resultant development of constipation. Once this sequence of events develops into a habit, it is difficult to break and lifelong constipation can result.

Some people will notice the onset of constipation in the middle-age years. The cause of constipation developing at this time is usually related to a change in dietary habits, decreased fluid intake, and the increasing inactivity of this age group. People in this age group may have medical illness that contributes to their constipation. They may be taking medications for these illnesses that have a side effect of constipation.

What illnesses and medications can result in constipation? The number of Americans taking medications regularly is increasing each year. Certain of these drugs will have a tendency to cause constipation. Fluid or water pills, which many patients with high blood pressure and heart failure take, may cause constipation by decreasing the water content within the large bowel and in the stool. Certain antacids, namely the calcium- and aluminum-containing preparations, will with regular usage result in a constipated state. Various drugs taken for the treatment of neurologic diseases will result in bowel irregularity. Medications taken for the treatment of seizures, depression, anxiety, Parkinson's disease, and muscle spasms may result in constipation. Iron, a mineral taken by many of us within our vitamin preparations, may cause bowel irregularity in certain individuals. Strong pain relievers, especially Codeine and other opiate derivatives, can result in constipation with their regular usage.

The list is longer, but now you are at least aware of the effect that certain medications may have on your bowel habits. Therefore, if constipation results after the regular usage of a drug, consult your physician to see if your constipation may be related to the drug or the illness for which the medication was prescribed.

Various disease states can also affect the regular functioning of the bowel. Diabetes, the type requiring insulin usage of long duration, may produce bowel irregularity secondary to its effects of the nerves to the digestive tract. People suffering from chronic renal failure may notice the onset of constipation. Hypothyroidism, the state of below-normal functioning of our thyroid gland, will result in a tendency toward constipation. Women during pregnancy routinely notice problems with constipation. Certain neurological diseases, especially those associated with paralysis of the legs, may result in bowel irregularity. It is easily seen that the interrelationships between various disease states and bowel function can result in a change in bowel habits in certain individuals.

It is important that persistent constipation occurring in any age group be evaluated by your physician. This is especially true of constipation developing in a middle-aged individual. Constipation alone or alternating with diarrhea, constipation associated with blood in the toilet bowl or mixed with the stools, or constipation occurring with stools of smaller caliber, all require prompt medical evaluation. All of the above symptoms could potentially be related to a tumor or cancer of the large bowel. I repeat, prompt medical evaluation of all persistent or newly recognized constipation is sound medical practice. Only in this way will an early tumor of the bowel be found. Fortunately, most people being evaluated for constipation will not be found to have a tumor as the cause of their constipation. Their constipation will result from an abnormal functioning of the large bowel.

Treatment of Constipation

Once an important medical cause of the constipation has been excluded, what is the treatment of known functional constipation? Adequate hydration, drinking enough fluids daily, is an important first step. The fluids allow the bowel contents to have proper hydration, which will facilitate easier passage through the large intestine. People who have their constipation on the basis of poor hydration frequently notice small, dry little balls of stool material. Many people with the "rabbit pellet stools" will notice lessening of their constipation with adequate fluid intake.

Once adequate hydration is achieved, dietary changes can be made in an attempt to relieve constipation. The consumption of a high-fiber diet will add bulk to the bowel movements and increase frequency of bowel movements. The fiber may be consumed in different breakfast cereals, in high-fiber or whole grain breads, selected vegetables with a high roughage content, and certain whole or stewed fruits. Some individuals find dietary fiber supplementing most easily accomplished by taking high-fiber bulk laxatives. These laxatives are made from natural vegetable fibers that have been ground up into a fine powder. A teaspoonful of these commercially available preparations is added to a glass of water or juice, once or twice daily. Millions of individuals have benefited from their regular usage. Your pharmacist will be happy to discuss these preparations with you. They vary greatly in taste, color, and acceptance among individuals. The pharmacist will help you find the right fiber supplement that your system will accept.

A four- to eight-week dietary trial is the first step in the treatment of functional constipation. While the dietary trial is underway, all individuals should be encouraged to increase their physical activity. This is especially true for middle-aged individuals. It is hoped that increased physical activity will stimulate the activity of the large bowel. The increased bowel activity, coupled with the increased bulk of the stool, will facilitate more regular bowel movements. During this trial, laxatives and enemas should not be used in an attempt to achieve normal functioning of the large bowel. It is impossible to predict accurately which individuals will respond to this approach. In my experience, the people with constipation of recent onset are more likely to respond than those suffering from constipation of many years' duration.

Another important practice is the regular habit of sitting on the commode at the same time daily. Many prefer the time after the evening meal when the calm allows time to read the newspaper. This is also a good time according to medical reasoning, for each of us has a normal reflex to have a bowel movement after eating a large meal. This daily habit may help in the reinstitution of a daily movement. Do not be discouraged early in this regard. Initially you might not have the urge to have a bowel movement. However, bowel retraining is an important factor in the resolution of persistent constipation. Persistence in this regard may be very rewarding.

For those individuals who fail to respond to the aforementioned treatment suggestions, a nonprescription stool softener should be added. The variety of stool softeners is endless, as you will notice in your drugstore. The response to various stool softeners will vary among individuals. A one- to two-week time trial is required to fully evaluate your response to each stool softener. A shorter time period is not adequate to determine your body's response to this medication.

If we are still troubled with constipation after the addition of a stool softener, the addition of a laxative compound containing a stool softener should then be tried. It is important when choosing a laxative to start with the mildest form of laxative first. The nonprescription laxatives are of approximately equal effectiveness. Again, an individual's response will vary greatly with usage of different laxatives. After regular bowel function has been present for a two- to four-week time period, the laxative should be discontinued. It is important now that we continue with the stool softener and dietary measures. If this is the case, the stool softener is then slowly withdrawn from usage. In this manner, some individuals will finally achieve bowel regularity without the need for stool softeners or laxatives. Others will require the addition of a stool softener and the intermittent use of a laxative for bowel regularity.

Certain individuals are less fortunate, however. The

habitual usage of certain laxatives for long periods of time could result in the development of a cathartic colon. This condition results from the habitual use of irritant laxatives over a period of more than fifteen years.[3] Laxatives described as irritant cathartics include those containing cascara, senna, resins such as podophyllin, oil preparations such as castor oil, or phenophthalin containing laxatives. The large intestine becomes thinned with poor motility or intestinal movement. In effect, the large intestine becomes an ineffective contracting, floppy structure.[4] Bowel movements may be only obtained with enema usage. Most importantly, the regular usage of soapsuds enemas is to be strongly discouraged. Although rarely, soapsuds enemas can produce a severe inflammation of the colon that might require surgery.

Other possible problems with habitual laxative usage include the possible aspiration or inadvertent passage of the oil into the lungs with a resultant pneumonia. If oil-containing laxatives are used, do not take them immediately before going to bed or lying down. The recumbent state may predispose to aspiration. Hypokalemia, or the state of a low body potassium level, is a frequent complication of continuous laxative usage. The lack of potassium results from the bowel secreting this substance into the fecal material. A low body potassium can result in muscular weakness, not only of our arms and legs, but also of the muscles within the intestine. Therefore, the hypokalemia may increase the constipation. Potentially serious problems can result from the lack of potassium for the normal functioning of the heart and kidneys.

It is easily seen that regular usage of laxatives is to be strongly discouraged. Use common sense in regard to laxative usage; for if you don't, the consequences may be severe.

Fecal impactions are a serious consequence of severe constipation, usually occurring in elderly people. These individuals are predisposed to fecal impactions due to their sedentary ways, altered dietary intake and associated medical conditions. Arthritis may make walking difficult, a stroke would make eating and having a bowel movement a difficult task, and forgetfulness tends to make food ingestion irregular. It is imperative that these individuals pay strict attention to their bowel function to prevent a fecal impaction.

Is there any medical evidence that prolonged constipation is harmful? Interestingly enough, there seems to be good evidence that constipation may be detrimental to good health. Studies have shown that both men and women who have a history of constipation have a higher incidence of cancer of the large bowel than those without a history of constipation.[5,6,7] Some authorities have difficulty accepting the fact that constipation could predispose individuals to cancer development. However, recent evidence shows that people with more rapid movement of food through the digestive tract have less cancer of the large bowel, or colon. It is hypothesized that the rate of cancer is lower because potential cancer substances are exposed to the lining of the large bowel for a shorter time period.

Proponents of the high-fiber diet can show that in countries where people regularly consume a high-fiber diet, there is a lower rate of colon cancer. The high-fiber diet results in a more rapid transit of food through the digestive tract. There would be less time for potential cancer causing agents to be exposed to the large bowel; therefore, a lower rate of cancer is indicated. Studies comparing the rate of cancer of the large bowel among Americans who consume a high-fiber diet for prolonged time periods with the cancer rate among those who have a low-fiber diet are presently underway. It will be many years before a final conclusion can be reached. All are hopeful that these results will be encouraging. In the meantime the consumption of a high-fiber diet surely can do no harm to the digestive system.

Summary

Bowel irregularity is a common occurrence among Americans. Most cases of constipation result from a functional cause. It is hoped that the suggestions outlined within this chapter will be of help to those with bowel irregularity. Importantly whenever blood is noticed within the bowel movements and there is associated constipation, contact your physician immediately.

chapter six

Diverticulosis and Diverticulitis

By definition, a diverticulum is an abnormal pouch or sac opening from a hollow organ, such as the large intestine. Therefore, diverticulosis is a condition in which the large intestine or colon has many saclike pouches protruding from its lining. These pouches, diverticula, are actually portions of the lining of the large intestine that have protruded through the colon's surrounding muscular wall. Colonic diverticulosis is a disease that is found most frequently with the advancing age of the individual. That is, this is a disease of older individuals. About one third of individuals over the age of sixty will have colonic diverticulosis.[1] Therefore, this is a disease that affects millions of Americans.

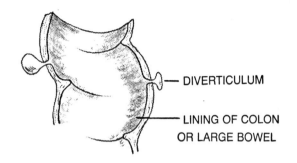

DIVERTICULUM

LINING OF COLON
OR LARGE BOWEL

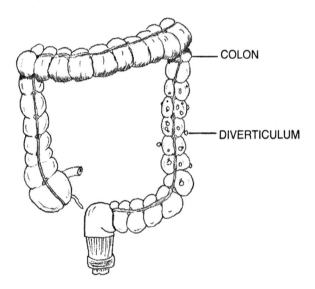

COLON

DIVERTICULUM

ILLUSTRATION 4. Diverticulosis.

Causes of Diverticula

Why do certain individuals develop colonic diverticula? Most authorities agree that people develop diverticula on the basis of abnormal bowel contractions or motility.[2] These abnormal contractions, or spasms of the large intestine, generate zones of high pressure within the organ. These high-pressure areas force the lining of the large intestine through weakened points in the bowel wall. Diverticula are thus formed and remain a permanent feature in these individuals. However, the experts cannot agree on the cause of this abnormal colonic motility.

Dietary fiber content has received much press recently regarding its possible role in the prevention of colonic diverticula formation. The enthusiasm for fiber content of our diet results from studies that have been conducted on the citizens of underdeveloped nations.[3,4] These carefully done studies have shown these individuals to have a low rate of occurrence of diverticulosis. The incidence of occurrence is lower than that observed in more industrialized nations. Concurrent with this lower incidence of diverticulosis is the observed higher dietary fiber intake of the citizens of the underdeveloped countries. Digestive disease experts feel that the additional bulk in the large intestine, supplied by the high-fiber diet, reduces the presssures that can be generated within the contracting large intestine. With the resultant decreased pressure within the large intestine, fewer diverticula are formed.

In countries with advanced industrialization techniques, there is more refinement in the preparation of food.[5] This processing of food usually results in a lower fiber content. The resultant lower bulk content of the diet results in a lower bulk residue in the large intestine and renders it more susceptible to diverticula formation.

Recent studies of people living in urbanized Africa reveal an incidence of occurrence of diverticulosis paralleling that seen in Americans.[6] This is more evidence to support the hypothesis that a high-fiber diet is important in the prevention of colonic diverticulosis.

Other digestive disease experts are not totally convinced that dietary fiber is the lone factor responsible for diverticular formation. They feel that other socioeconomic factors are responsible for the observed difference in the occurrence of diverticular disease among individuals in underdeveloped and industrialized countries. They hypothesize that the difference in social standards and the number of stressful situations are equally as important as dietary fiber. Individuals living in a more industrialized country will be exposed more often to stressful situations because of the demands of their social and economic environment. Studies have shown that the large intestine is capable of generating extremely high pressures when an individual is placed in a stressful situation.[7] This observation lends support to the idea that diverticula formation can be related to stress.

These experts state that the difference in social customs may be an important consideration in explaining the difference in occurrence of diverticular disease.[8] In underdeveloped countries, social customs permit flatulence and defecation in any accessible area. These social habits allow pressure within the large intestine to be reduced immediately. In industrialized countries social habits prohibit flatulence and require the usage of lavatory facilities. Because these facilities are sometimes inaccessible, the large intestine can be exposed to periods of increased pressure for long intervals. Regardless of the exact reason, we and our large intestines pay the price for our cultural and industrial development.

Symptoms of Colonic Diverticulosis

What are the symptoms of colonic diverticulosis? There are no specific symptoms related to the presence of diverticula within the colon. Most individuals have this diagnosis made when a barium enema examination is being performed to exclude some other medical condition. Some individuals with diverticulosis will demonstrate an intolerance of high-roughage food substances. They will complain of bloating and crampy abdominal pains after the ingestion of popcorn, nuts, and seed-containing foods. The exact reason why these high-roughage foods produce such symptoms in these individuals is not fully understood.

Treatment
of Colonic Diverticulosis

What is the treatment of colonic diverticulosis? Formerly, individuals known to have colonic diverticula were advised to consume a low-residue diet. With the recent evidence regarding the usage of a high-fiber diet in the prevention of intestinal diverticula formation, many individuals are now being treated with a high-fiber diet. Some of these people will be able to tolerate this high-bulk diet, while others will find that their symptoms of bloating and crampy abdominal pains are increased with its usage. In those intolerant individuals it is important to stop the diet despite the encouragement of their family or physician. Your body knows what is right for it.

To my thinking, once a person has diverticulosis, it is too late for the high-fiber diet to be beneficial. Regular ingestion of a high-fiber diet is required from youth to prevent the formation of diverticula. The sudden usage of a high-fiber diet, once the intestinal diverticula have formed, may produce uncomfortable and unnecessary symptoms.

If you have diverticulosis, you will know your body's acceptance of such a diet soon after its institution. If the diet produces no symptoms, I would recommend its continued usage, not for the prevention of further diverticular formation, but rather for its bulk laxative effect. Bowel regularity is an important habit for patients with colonic diverticulosis to maintain. Constipation should be avoided. A high-fiber or residue diet, if acceptable by the patient's intestinal tract, is an excellent foundation of a program for bowel regularity.

To facilitate bowel regularity, patients with diverticulosis should maintain regular physical activity, drink an adequate amount of fluid, and use a stool softener as needed for the prevention of constipation.

Can Diverticulitis Be Prevented?

Does the treatment of diverticulosis prevent attacks of acute inflammation of the diverticula, or acute diverticulitis? There are no medical studies to prove or disprove that treatment of diverticulosis is effective in the prevention of the development of diverticulitis. It is hoped that results of the ongoing clinical studies will answer this question. Presently treatment suggestions for colonic diverticulosis should be used to prevent individuals from having recurrent symptoms of abdominal pain or bloating.

Usually, harsh laxatives or irritant laxatives are not tolerated well by people with extensive diverticulosis. These laxatives may result in severe spasm of the intestine and crampy abdominal pain. I am hopeful that the dietary alterations and the intermittent usage of bowel softeners will prevent the need for laxative usage in these individuals.

Complications of Colonic Diverticulosis

Are there any complications of colonic diverticulosis? Diverticulitis is the most frequent and important complication of diverticulosis. Diverticulitis is an inflammation of multiple diverticula in a short segment of the large intestine. Acute diverticulitis develops in approximately 10 to 25 percent of individuals with colonic diverticulosis.[9] Diverticulitis is more likely to occur in individuals having a large number of colonic diverticula.

Causes and Symptoms
of Diverticulitis

What causes a diverticulum to become inflamed? Why does diverticulitis occur? No one knows with certainty, but theories suggest that the opening of the diverticulum becomes blocked, with subsequent infection of the diverticula. What causes the block of the opening of the diverticula is certain. It is indeed possible that certain undigested foods such as nuts, popcorn, and seed-containing foods could block the opening. This is another reason why these foods should be restricted in individuals known to have colonic diverticulosis.

Individuals experiencing an attack of acute diverticulitis will usually have severe abdominal pain with associated fever. The pain is usually located in the lower left side of the abdomen. The pain is located in this area, for this is the portion of the intestine that has the greatest number of diverticula, and therefore the greatest incidence of diverticular inflammation. The pain may be so severe that the individual will have to walk bent over. Occasionally pain will be made worse with this walking or any movement of the abdominal cavity. Not infrequently, there will be associated chills with the fever. Shaking chills, "teeth-rattling chills," can occur in individuals with acute diverticulitis. Although it rarely occurs, an individual may have only the fever and chills without any abdominal pain. In both situations the individual will feel sick enough to consult a physician.

Treatment of Diverticulitis

The treatment of acute diverticulitis usually requires hospitalization. The large intestine will be rested by the drainage of the stomach and intestinal secretions that could stimulate the large intestine. This drainage will be accomplished by the placement of a tube through the nose into the stomach. The tube is then connected to a suction machine that will drain the unwanted contents. Fluids will be taken in through a vein to supply the needed fluid and nutrient requirements. Antibiotics are usually given to combat the inflammation and infection. Most individuals will respond to some form of this therapy and be ready for discharge within a week. Unfortunately, these inflamed diverticula frequently breakdown because of the inflammation. Remember that a diverticulum is only as thin as the lining of the large intestine. If the infected and inflamed diverticulum ruptures, complications occur. A collection of the inflammatory pus could collect around the large intestine. This collection of pus could block the outflow from the large intestine. In this case individuals would notice difficulty having a bowel movement. If the bowel blockage was severe enough, an individual would notice inability to have any bowel movement.

The ruptured diverticulum may erode into the urinary system, the female organs, or the small intestine. This erosion could result in a connection, called a fistula, between the large intestine and these organs. A fistula to the urinary system could result in a urinary infection or the passage of air in the urinary stream. A fistula, or connection, between the large intestine and the female organs could result in a vaginal discharge and the passage of fecal material through the vagina. If any of these complications occurred, as a result of the rupture of an inflamed diverticula, surgery would usually be necessary to correct the problem.

Bleeding from the Diverticulum

Another complication of diverticulosis is bleeding from the diverticulum. Bleeding from a diverticulum occurs in up to a third of individuals with colonic diverticulosis. If bleeding does occur from the diverticulum, acute inflammation or acute diverticulitis is not required for this bleeding to occur. Usually, the bleeding rate would be slow with intermittent spotting of blood noted within the bowel movement. Severe bleeding, or hemorrhage, occurs in about one in twenty individuals experiencing a bleeding episode from colonic diverticulosis.[10] The colonic bleeding is painless and not associated with chills or fever. Bleeding from colonic diverticular disease stops spontaneously in the majority of the cases. Unfortunately, once an individual has experienced a bleeding episode from their diverticula, they have a 25 percent chance of re-bleeding.[11] Surgery may be required for these individuals with bleeding that is profuse, uncontrollable, or recurrent and results in severe anemia. Surgery, however, is only required in about 10 percent of all cases.[12]

Summary

In summary, millions of Americans have diverticular disease of their large intestine. Most suffer only from diverticulosis. The dietary approach to the treatment of colonic diverticulosis has been reviewed. All patients will not be able to tolerate a high-fiber diet. The maintenance of bowel regularity in the prevention of constipation is important. Diverticulitis is the acute inflammation of a colonic diverticulum. Diverticulitis has many serious complications that are fortunately rare in occurrence. Whether a high-fiber diet will prevent individuals in this country from developing colonic diverticulosis remains to be determined by ongoing medical studies.

chapter seven

Spastic Colon, Mucous Colitis, or the Irritable Bowel Syndrome

These three medical terms are synonymous for a very commonly occurring medical condition. Between 30 to 40 million Americans have been diagnosed as having this digestive tract disease. However, probably more than 100 million individuals suffer, at least intermittently, from some form of this digestive disease. This entity has been reported to account for one third of all patient visits to all physicians interested in digestive tract diseases.[1] This condition also has a great economic impact on the American economy. Dr. Thomas Almy, presently professor of medicine at the Dartmouth Medical School, has studied this disease extensively. His studies demonstrated that in 1967, this condition ranked behind the common cold as a reason why people missed work.[2] The magnitude of this medical condition has not really been fully appreciated. However, through the efforts of individuals such as Dr. Thomas Almy, we are beginning to understand the importance of this condition.

This digestive tract disease results from the abnormal motility within the intestinal tract. This abnormal motility is frequently associated with spasms within the digestive system. Importantly, there is no evidence for any inflammation within the intestines. The term *colitis* implies an inflammation of the large bowel. Therefore, this term should not be used when desribing this condition. The term *colitis* only serves to confuse the individuals suffering with this condition.

Not infrequently patients say that their having colitis is the reason they have come to be evaluated by me. However, after interviewing them, it becomes apparent that there is no evidence for colonic inflammation, or colitis; rather, they are suffering from the spastic colon or the irritable bowel syndrome. I prefer these descriptive terms for this condition because they eliminate confusion with any inflammatory bowel disease and they help explain the reason for the patient's symptoms.

This digestive disease has been shown to have a definite relationship to the emotional status of those individuals afflicted. Clearly, most individuals are aware of the coincidental relationships of their bowel symptoms to periods in their life where there is increased tension or stress. "Doc, I am worse when I am nervous." "My job is wrecking my bowel habits." These are frequent descriptions that people relate to explain the interrelationship of their bowel symptoms and their emotional states.

Tension and the Spastic Colon Syndrome

Why and how does tension cause the spastic colon syndrome? All of us have different methods in which our body handles the emotional tensions to which we are exposed. Our body reacts to lower the tension to a level that we can tolerate. Some people notice sweating, flushing of the face, and sweaty palms when "under the gun." Others will experience acid indigestion. Some will feel the urgency for frequent urination. Certain individuals will hyperventilate, that is, breathe deeper and more rapidly than normal. This process occurs unconsciously and can result in lightheadness, shortness of breath, chest pains, and a sensation of "pins and needles" in the hands and around the mouth. A few individuals will feel a sensation of fullness in their throat, which makes them constantly clear their throat. All of us have either experienced one or more of these tension-relieving methods or have noticed our friends reacting in one of these ways. All of these mechanisms are means by which our body reduces life's stresses and strains to an acceptable level.

People who are predisposed to have an irritable bowel utilize their large intestine as the method of decreasing tension. Their large bowel absorbs, so to speak, the brunt of their problems. Their bowel function is in shambles, but they look calm and collected. Studies have shown that these individuals, when put in stressful situations, exhibit abnormal bowel function and motility.[3,4] This abnormal bowel motility and function produces the symptoms of the spastic colon syndrome.

People suffering from an irritable bowel syndrome complain of varying symptoms. Abdominal pain, a pressured or crampy pain, occurs in the lower left and right portions of the abdomen. This pain is usually worse one to two hours after eating and may be relieved by either a bowel movement or the passage of intestinal gas. Many individuals experiencing this abdominal pain will also note abdominal bloating.

Some people describe a discomfort occurring in the left upper part of the abdomen. This pain may radiate under the left rib cage, into the left side of the chest, and into the left axilla, or armpit. This pain may closely resemble cardiac pain, and many individuals experiencing this pain feel they are having a heart attack. Prudently many seek medical evaluation and may even be admitted to an intensive care unit for the exclusion of a heart attack. This pain syndrome is known as the splenic flexure syndrome.[5] It results from the gaseous distension and spasms of the large intestine, which lies beneath the left rib cage and is known as the splenic flexure portion of the large bowel. This specific condition can occur in any age group. I recommend to all people experiencing the previously described pain to seek prompt medical advice so that a heart attack can be excluded. Remember, some sufferers of the spastic colon syndrome also have heart disease.

Individuals with the irritable bowel syndrome will complain of abdominal bloating or swelling of the abdomen. Typically these symptoms occur a couple of hours after eating. Not uncommonly, individuals have the sensation of things moving within their distended abdomen. All of these symptoms are related to the fluid and gas-filled large bowel, which has problems propelling its contents normally. As previously stated, this is due to the abnormal bowel motility. Importantly the above symptoms are also helped by the passage of intestinal gas or having a bowel movement.

Constipation is another frequent complaint of people suffering from an irritable bowel experience. The abnormal motilty of the large bowel predisposes the individual to bowel irregularity and constipation. The spasms of the large intestine allow for a slower passage of the stool material, which results in larger quantities of water being removed. Therefore, people with constipation, as a symptom of their irritable bowel, frequently notice "rabbit pellet stools."[6]

Most individuals with an irritable bowel notice diarrhea which may alternate with periods of constipation. Some sufferers experience only diarrhea and hope or wish for periods of constipation. Typically, the diarrhea occurs upon awakening in the morning. This may necessitate two or three sittings in the lavatory before breakfast can be eaten. Not uncommonly, immediately after eating breakfast, another one to two movements may occur. This pattern is very typical of most patients with diarrhea associated with an irritable bowel syndrome.

Individuals may notice semi-formed loose stools with the first movement of the day. Subsequent bowel movements contain less and less fecal material. Patients will notice mucoid whitish material in their bowel movements. Sometimes, individuals pass only this mucous material upon having the sensation of rectal urgency. The diarrhea and the mucoid material results from the altered bowel motility and increased bowel secretions in this syndrome. Importantly, the mucoid material does not indicate infection or inflammation within the intestine.

Another feature of the diarrhea associated with the irritable bowel syndrome is that it rarely occurs after the individual has fallen asleep. This feature helps to separate it from the diarrhea occurring with an inflammatory bowel disease. Diarrhea associated with either ulcerative colitis or Crohn's disease may awaken the individual many times during the night. Also, the diarrhea associated with a spastic colon never contains blood, as that of a person with inflammatory bowel disease.

Another symptom experienced by many persons with an irritable colon is the urgency to have a bowel movement soon after eating. This occurs most frequently after breakfast and supper. This rectal urgency results from an increased or heightened normal occurring reflex. This gastrocolic reflex results in the feeling of the need to have a bowel movement approximately one hour after eating. In individuals with the irritable bowel syndrome, this reflex is greatly enhanced, resulting in true rectal urgency soon after eating.[7]

Because of what I have described, it is not unusual for some patients with a spastic colon to have six to ten bowel movements daily. The majority of them will occur early in the morning before leaving for work. This frequency of trips to the bathroom necessitates a great change in life style. Some patients have related how it is almost impossible to go shopping for long periods of time because of the constant fear of needing a restroom nearby. Their efficiency at work may suffer, and some bosses are not the most understanding about all those bathroom breaks. Truly, the irritable bowel syndrome may make a lot of different people irritable besides those unfortunate individuals suffering with it.

A very unfortunate thing happens to many individuals suffering with a tension-related colon syndrome. Many are told that their symptoms are only in their head. This situation results because of the nervous character of many of these individuals and the busy time schedules of their physicians. The doctor does not have the time or the desire to explain to these individuals why they are having their problems. However, it is obvious to anyone who is sitting on a toilet ten times a day that this symptom does not exist in his or her head. The abdominal pain that these individuals experience is real and results from the abnormal intestinal motility. When time is taken to explain to these unfortunate individuals the causes of their abdominal pain, the majority are relieved to know that there is a physiological rather than a psychological cause. They are truly grateful for the extra time spent in describing the interrelationship of their symptoms and their anxiety-tension level.

Many individuals work hard and are effective in changing their body's mechanisms of handling life's tensions. These people are able to reduce the severity and frequency of the symptoms of their irritable bowel. They are able to function more effectively at work and in our society. The additional time and effort spent by the patient and physician may be very rewarding.

Breaking the Stress–Spastic Colon Cycle

How are some individuals able to break the stress–spastic colon cycle? First the realization that there is no true serious illness producing their symptoms gives mental relief to many. Then they must work hard to recognize the situations and emotional stresses that cause their symptoms. When a similar situation occurs, they must make a conscious effort to use another mechanism to cope with this situation. They may talk over the situation or make mental changes in attitude to perceive the problem differently. An honest, hard effort in this regard may yield dramatic results in breaking the stress–spastic colon cycle.

Some individuals suffering with an irritable bowel syndrome will require medication to assist them in breaking the stress–spastic colon cycle. Minor tranquilizers are often helpful to lower the anxiety level of these selected patients to a degree where they are able to cope with their emotions. Once the individual is more settled, he or she can proceed with the personality changes necessary for a more efficient handling of his or her emotional state. Because of the ease with which these minor tranquilizers can be obtained, some people use them as a long-standing crutch when dealing with life's pressures. These drugs should not be used in all individuals with a spastic colon syndrome. It is my opinion that these medications are used on too wide a scale with this digestive syndrome.

Breaking the stress-symptom cycle will take time. Do not get impatient with yourself. Especially, do not get disappointed. This could reverse any gain that you may have made in breaking the cycle. Truly, patience is a virtue with this condition.

Most patients with the irritable bowel syndrome will benefit from a bowel relaxant. This bowel relaxant will help decrease the abnormal intestinal motility and spasms. Many patients respond favorably to these bowel relaxants, or antispasmodics, as they are known. They will notice a decrease in their diarrhea, a decrease in their rectal urgency, and will experience less abdominal pain. Their bloating and gaseous state will also improve. People with constipation as a symptom of their tension-related colon syndrome do not respond as favorably to these medications. In fact, their constipation may be made worse.

The bowel relaxants can gradually be reduced in the majority of patients as they gain more effectiveness in dealing with the stress-symptom cycle. These medications should be given only as a part of the total approach to the patient's problem. Unfortunately, many times they are given without an explanation to the patient of the basic reason behind the symptoms. In those patients the results may not be as good as when time was taken to outline the etiology of their symptoms. It is important to stress the need for a change in mental attitude when approaching stressful situations.

Many patients with an irritable bowel notice help from the addition of a high-fiber diet alone, or in combination with bulk laxatives. The additional bulk in the large intestine reduces the pressures that can be generated within it. Therefore, their abdominal pains should be less and the bulk residue would help solidify their bowel movements. Surprisingly, the same combination may facilitate more regular bowel movements in those with constipation. Each treatment program must be individualized for the specific needs of each patient.

Now, you sufferers of the tension-related colon syndrome can realize how important your role is in preventing the recurrence of your symptoms. Don't rely entirely on medications. Help break the stress-symptom cycle with effort, willingness, and patience.

It is hoped that your friends and employers will now recognize and understand the disease from which you suffer. It is so common in today's society. Their understanding and help may allow many more people to break the stress-symptom cycle.

Remember, the daily pressures that we are all under may result in troublesome pressures within the large intestine.

chapter eight

Lactose
Intolerance

Lactose intolerance is a frequent cause of digestive symptoms in Americans. Millions of Americans are intolerant to the sugar in milk and milk products.[1] This disease entity results from their inability to absorb the milk sugar called lactose. The undigested sugar is acted upon by bacteria within the large bowel and the products that result from this reaction produce the digestive tract symptoms.

Diarrhea, abdominal cramps, bloating, or abdominal distension and flatulence are frequent symptoms individuals with lactose intolerance notice after the ingestion of milk or milk products. The abdominal bloating and flatulence are related to the gases that are produced as a result of the bacterial reaction with the unabsorbed milk sugar. The diarrhea results from the large quantities of water that enter the large intestine to counterbalance the presence of the excess sugars there. Certain acids, produced by the bacterial action on the undigested milk sugar, stimulate the large intestine and contribute to the resultant diarrhea.

Causes of Lactose Intolerance

There is a definite racial and ethnic predilection for developing lactose intolerance. Medical statistics show that somewhere between 40 to 90 percent of black and Chinese Americans will be intolerant to milk.[2,3] About two thirds of American Jews and American Indians will demonstrate lactose intolerance.[4,5] Close to 10 percent of Caucasian Americans will be unable to tolerate milk or milk products.[6,7] How the racial or ethnic composition of an individual is responsible for the development of the lactose intolerance is unknown. It is known that individuals suffering from this condition will continue to demonstrate this intolerance despite geographical movement. Therefore, environmental factors are not important determinants of this condition.

Lactose intolerance most often develops in adults who have had no prior history of problems with milk ingestion.[8] This intolerance may develop suddenly in some individuals, with others noticing a gradual unacceptance of milk or milk products. The reason why some adults suddenly cannot tolerate milk is unknown.

Sometimes while interviewing a patient in regard to his or her dietary history, the patient will relate avoidance of milk or milk products for years. These individuals have recognized their intolerance of the milk sugar and have changed their diet accordingly to prevent the occurrence of symptoms. Some individuals, thought to have an irritable bowel syndrome because of their symptoms of bloating, crampy pains, and diarrhea, are now being recognized as having their symptoms because of lactose intolerance.[9] Both of these digestive diseases are very frequent among Americans. Some unfortunate individuals will actually have both diseases.

Some children become intolerant to the sugar in milk. Usually, this milk intolerance is noticed between the ages of three to five. Children will more commonly experience bloating and crampy abdominal pains than diarrhea. Therefore, lactose intolerance may be a cause of colic in preschool children. This may be another reason why children stop drinking milk at this time. The parents' failure to understand their children's reason and their concern that the children receive the known benefits of milk may cause a ticklish family situation. An important clue may be the child's sudden disliking of ice cream. When a three- to four-year-old suddenly refuses an ice cream cone you know something is wrong. Listen to your children, for they are trying to tell you something that is important to them. However, most children will decrease their milk intake during these years because of the development of new tastes rather than on the basis of lactose intolerance.

Most Americans who are intolerant of milk are so because of their ethnic or racial predisposition to be so. Only rarely will milk intolerance be the first sign of another digestive disease.[10] These diseases cause the small intestine to be unable to take up the milk sugar properly. Some patients recovering from a viral gastroenteritis will notice that they have become milk intolerant. This milk intolerance will usually last a couple of weeks, but in some may last up to six months. Some people with ulcerative colitis or Crohn's disease will be intolerant to milk. Some ulcer patients will notice the development of milk intolerance after they have had an ulcer operation. This results from a change in the flow pattern within their digestive tract. The milk arrives sooner and less digested so that the small intestine cannot handle it properly.

Lactose intolerance is easily diagnosed if a clear cut relationship is established between milk ingestion and the development of symptoms. In some individuals the cause of abdominal bloating and diarrhea will be correctly diagnosed only if this common condition is thought of by the physician.

Remember that lactose intolerance and an irritable bowel can occur in some unfortunate individuals.

A simple test can confirm the presence or absence of lactose intolerance. During this test a person will drink a glass of milk or a mixture of lactose sugar. Blood samples are then drawn at the half hour and thereafter at hourly intervals for up to five hours. The person is questioned about any symptoms that he or she notices that are identical to those that occur after drinking a glass of milk or consuming milk products. If the symptoms are reproduced, then a positive test is noted and the diagnosis of lactose intolerance is established. If no symptoms occur, the correct diagnosis can still be etablished from the results of the blood samples.

The Relationship of Diet to Lactose Intolerance

Once the diagnosis of lactose intolerance is made, the patient can experience relief of the symptoms by simply restricting his or her milk intake. Some individuals will notice relief through a simple reduction in the amount of milk or milk products they ingest. Other individuals will require a completely milk-free diet before they notice any improvement. Remember that milk is in many good things that we eat daily and take for granted. Breads, cookies, sauces, and creams, and many other goodies contain milk. Individuals requiring a totally milk-free diet must severely alter their food intake.

A new product can help such individuals liberalize their diets. Lact-Aid is this new product. Lact-Aid is added to a quart of milk and then the milk is allowed to sit in the refrigerator. This substance changes the milk sugar so that the individuals can now tolerate it. They can now drink this milk and cook with it. Breads, cakes and cookies, mayonnaise, puddings—all the good things—can now be made and eaten. The only noticeable difference between Lact-Aid-treated milk and regular milk is that the treated milk has a slightly sweeter taste. Lact-Aid-prepared milk is now available in some grocery stores in certain areas of the United States. If Lact-Aid-prepared milk is not commercially available to you, consult your physician for information regarding its purchase. A distinct type of milk intolerance occurs in certain infants. All of us have known babies that could not tolerate cows' milk and had to be raised on soybean milk.[11] Fortunately, most of these infants can, as they grow older, drink regular milk. This condition results from the infant's intestine not having the ability to break down the milk sugar properly. This inability is overcome with age in most cases.

Summary

Milk, that wonderful food substance on which we were all raised, can sometimes turn its back on us. The intolerance to milk sugar may result in bloating, crampy pains, and diarrhea in those unfortunate individuals. If you experience the aforementioned symptoms, try to establish a relationship between your symptoms and the ingestion of milk or milk products. In most individuals a simple alteration of diet will result in improvement. If your symptoms persist despite these dietary changes, consult your physician in this regard.

chapter nine

Diarrhea

Diarrhea is a frequent cause of concern for millions of Americans. The crampy abdominal pains and the necessity for all those bathroom visits make this digestive symptom one of the most unpleasant to experience. This symptom necessitates many days away from school and dutiful employment.

Causes of Diarrhea

Diarrhea has multiple causes,[1] some of which we have already discussed, but the most frequent cause is a viral infection of the small intestine resulting in a viral gastroenteritis. This viral infection causes the intestine to secrete large quantities of water and salt, which results in the frequent, watery bowel movements. The stimulated intestine reacts with abnormal contractions and spasm that produce the crampy pains. The increased number of bowel movements and the water secreted by the intestine could result in a dehydrated state unless precautions are taken to prevent its occurrence. Most viral diarrheal illnesses last only a couple of days. During these most uncomfortable couple of days individuals will use different remedies to decrease their cramps and the number of trips they have to make to the bathroom. The first measure that the majority of individuals with diarrhea take is to change their dietary intake. They change their diet to consist of liquids only. The full liquid diet seems to produce less abdominal cramping and diarrhea. It is also important to prevent dehydration from occurring. Many individuals use clear soups or bouillons to help replace the salt and minerals they have lost through their diarrhea. There are also commercially available liquids that are high in varying salt content. Gatorade has been useful in many of my patients with viral gastroenteritis. Certainly the ingestion of a lot of caffein-containing liquid should be avoided. Caffeine is a known stimulant of the digestive tract.

Remedies for Diarrhea

There are as many different remedies for diarrhea as there are sufferers of diarrhea. Many individuals consume burnt toast with tea during their acute diarrheal illness. This approach to diarrhea has been passed down from generation to generation. The burnt layer of the toast is felt to contain charcoal and is the basis for this dietary maneuver. Charcoal has long been used in the treatment of digestive disorders. Today, it is still possible to buy charcoal preparations in the pharmacy to help in the treatment of various digestive symptoms such as diarrhea. Some families have long advocated the use of blackberry brandy for the control of abdominal cramps and diarrhea. Users of this remedy will attest to its effectiveness. Could it be that the influence of the brandy allows those individuals to be more tolerant of their intestinal cramps? Many sufferers of diarrhea use pectin-containing over-the-counter drugs for the control of their symptoms. Bismuth-containing antidiarrheal medications are another popular form of therapy. Pepto-Bismol, made by Eaton Laboratories, is the most widely known bismuth antidiarrheal drug. This form of treatment is advocated by some people having diarrhea.

Everyone will swear by his or her own form of therapy for controlling the symptoms of a viral gastroenteritis. People who try a suggested remedy may be disappointed with the results. Each of us must find his or her own combination that will make the "viral trots" more easy to live through.

Treating Diarrhea While Traveling

Traveler's diarrhea, tourista, or Montezuma's revenge are all names given to the explosive diarrheal illness that can occur during one's visit to sunny South America or Mexico.[2] If you are one of the unfortunate individuals to be afflicted with this, the only redness you may get during your vacation could be on your bottom because of the requirements for frequent wipings. This diarrheal illness has ruined many expensive vacations to many warm and sunny places.

Traveler's diarrhea results from a certain type of bacteria, called E. coli, which is found in the water of these countries. This bacteria results in an infection of the small intestine, which produces large quantities of water to be secreted with its resultant diarrhea. Travelers to Mexico are always warned about this illness and are instructed not to drink the water or use ice in their drinks. Unfortunately, you can develop tourista even if you follow these suggestions stringently. Remember that most salad greens and fruits are washed with water before being served. People have developed this illness from eating only these foods and not drinking the water. Certainly all of these restrictions can limit your sampling of all of the delicious South American or Mexican foods. This illness is associated with an explosive diarrhea that occurs at very frequent intervals. Many individuals have known the need to be restricted to their lodging accommodations because of the severity of the symptoms. What can you do once you become a victim of this revenge?[3] Some people will take an antidiarrheal prescription drug given to them by their doctors before leaving on their vacations. Medications such as Lomotil or Imodium are most frequently used in this regard. The majority of the time these medications will be less than totally effective and may make the abdominal cramping worse. These antidiarrheal medications do seem to shorten the duration of the illness by a couple of hours. The average length of symptoms associated with traveler's diarrhea, or Montezuma's revenge, is anywhere from twenty-four to forty-eight hours. Therefore, two to three hours of improvement may be welcome relief for those afflicted.

Pepto-Bismol has been used for some years in treating this acute diarrheal illness.[4] At the earliest sign of symptoms, an individual should take six to eight full bottles of this over-the-counter drug. This remedy has saved many vacations from being a total loss. One obvious drawback to this form of therapy is the large volume of medication that must be consumed. Another drawback is finding room for the bottles within your suitcases. A more serious drawback is the potential consequence of having six bottles of Pepto-Bismol spilled over your clothing. Despite these limitations this form of treatment for travelers diarrhea remains an acceptable approach for individuals afflicted with this digestive illness.

Can antibiotics be used to prevent tourista or Montezuma's revenge?[5] Many well-controlled studies have been performed on American medical students or physicians visiting these countries. Various antibiotics have been included within these studies. There are encouraging signs that some of the newer combination antibiotics may be helpful in the prevention or the control of symptoms if one is afflicted with this illness. Physicians as a whole have reacted differently to the results of these studies. Certain physicians will now give these antibiotics to be taken only if symptoms occur, while others will recommend the usage of these antibiotics to prevent symptoms. I can only recommend that you discuss this issue completely with your physician before leaving on your vacation to the sunny south.

A diarrheal illness can occur while traveling in any foreign country. These diarrheal illnesses usually result from various bacteria or parasites found within the drinking water.[6] These illnesses are again of short duration but severe in their symptoms. It is most important that if any diarrheal illness persists upon returning home, this symptom should be evaluated fully by your physician. An analysis of a stool specimen will be done to exclude any bacteria or parasitic cause for your persistent diarrhea. If such organisms are found during this evaluation, effective oral medications can rid the bacteria or parasitic organisms from your stool and result in the resolution of your symptoms.

Diarrhea Caused by Bacteria

Diarrhea caused by bacteria still occurs sporadically within the United States. The incidence of occurrence has decreased greatly with the advent of uniform water purification systems and the widespread usage of refrigeration. The bacteria most commonly causing a diarrheal illness within the United States are the Staphylococcus, Salmonella, Shigella, and Campylobacter organisms. The diarrheal state results from either the direct inflammatory effect of the bacteria on the intestinal tract or toxins that are produced by the bacteria, which stimulate the intestine to secrete fluids.

Staph food poisoning can result from the ingestion of outdated dairy or milk products or eating spoiled meats.[7] Typically an individual will eat a baked good filled with a cream sauce that has spoiled. Within two to four hours these individuals will notice the onset of nausea, vomiting, intestinal cramps, and diarrhea. These symptoms may last for twenty-four to thirty-six hours. After this time the individual will have a full recovery from the symptoms. I always try to let the bakery or restaurant know how their dessert was when I am afflicted with such symptoms.

A Shigella infection can result in a short diarrheal illness or in a full-blown bacterial dysentery state.[8] Bacillary dysentery is most commonly observed where conditions predispose to poor sanitary measures. This digestive tract illness is most commonly seen during war times or after natural catastrophies where the sanitary works are destroyed. Many of our war veterans can remember their buddies suffering with "the dysentery." The Shigella infections occurring within this country usually result from a fecal contamination of a water source or poor well water.

Bacillary dysentery is a fulminant diarrheal illness.[9] It is associated with bloody diarrhea, severe intestinal cramps, and signs of body toxicity such as fever, prostration, and a cloudy sensorium. Severe dehydration and shock can occur quickly unless appropriate measures are taken to prevent them. Some individuals will require up to thirty-two quarts of fluid during a forty-eight to seventy-two hour period for the prevention of dehydration and shock. This illness will usually last from four to seven days. Eventual recovery occurs without complications if dehydration is prevented.

Milder forms of Shigella infections may have nonbloody diarrhea and less findings of systemic toxicity from this bacterial infection of our intestinal tract. Recovery in four to seven days is the rule, but rarely, a chronic diarrheal state can result.

The Salmonella bacteria can cause a gastroenteritis characterized by nausea and vomiting, intestinal crampy pain, and diarrhea. This illness usually has a clinical course of three to five days. The correct diagnosis can easily be established by performing a stool analysis for the presence of the Salmonella bacteria. There are many different Salmonella bacterial organisms.[10] One specific Salmonella bacteria causes the commonly occurring Salmonella gastroenteritis. A different Salmonella bacteria causes typhoid fever. Therefore, people having a Salmonella gastroenteritis do not have to worry about developing typhoid fever. Individuals with sickle-cell anemia who develop a Salmonella infection may get a severe arthritis from this bacteria. This unusual cause of an arthritis can result in these individuals because the form of the red blood cell has somehow affected the body's inability to clear the Salmonella bacteria from the system. Importantly individuals not having sickle cell anemia rarely develop this form of arthritis.

The number one cause of a bacterial diarrheal illness within the United States today is due to an organism known as the Campylobacter bacteria.[11] The importance of this organism as a cause of diarrheal illness has only been recently recognized. This bacteria has long been known by our veterinary colleagues as a cause of various illnesses within animals. A most important fact is that our household pets such as dogs and cats are the natural reservoir for this organism. Unfortunately, our pets develop diarrhea as their owners do. Caring for our sick pets at such time and cleaning up their accidents allow for the exposure to this bacteria. This form of bacterial infection will result in either plain diarrhea or possibly bloody diarrhea. Because of the characteristics of this bacteria to inflame the intestines, this specific form of a bacterial gastroenteritis may mimic an ulcerative colitis or a Crohn's disease inflammation. Once again, this cause of a diarrheal illness can be easily established by the analysis of a stool sample. This form of a bacterial gastroenteritis can be easily treated with an Erythromycin form of an antibiotic.

Individuals may contract a diarrheal illness by eating seafood containing a certain Vibrio bacteria.[12] Crabmeat is the most common seafood contaminated with this organism. Groups of individuals eating the same crabmeat dish will notice the onset of diarrhea and crampy intestinal pains soon after the meal. This illness may last up to three days, but more commonly lasts only twenty-four hours. Complete recovery from this bacterial cause of diarrhea is the rule.

Giardia infections are increasing as a cause of diarrheal illness. This organism is an intestinal parasite that has a worldwide distribution. This infestation results from drinking water contaminated with the Giardia organism. Recently a large number of cases of Giardia infections have been reported occurring within the United States. Most commonly these have occurred in the mountainous areas of our country. People are flocking to these locales for skiing enjoyment or backpacking trips in the warmer months. The water in the pristine mountain streams can be contaminated with this parasite. Those of us living in low-lying areas of the United States are not spared from this cause of diarrhea. Giardia diarrhea has been reported in each state of the United States.

Infection by the Giardia organism can be prevented by disinfecting suspected drinking water by adding 12.5 ml. or cc. of a saturated iodine solution to each liter of water. This prepared water is safe for consumption after sitting for fifteen minutes.[13] This is a very important consideration for campers and hikers who will be visiting the inner regions of the American mountain chains.

Other Causes of Diarrhea

Diarrhea can occur as a manifestation of the irritable bowel syndrome. We have discussed this cause of diarrhea in Chapter 7. Certainly, all of us have experienced diarrhea when we have gotten nervous. Remember those loose bowel movements before that big game or your first date with your childhood sweetheart? That diarrhea resulted from our increased nervous tension. Some less fortunate individuals suffer daily from diarrhea because of problems in handling life's daily pressures.

Diarrhea may result from diseases other than those affecting the digestive system. Diarrhea may be the first and only symptom of a hyperfunctioning thyroid. A hyperthyroid state results from the overproduction of thyroid hormone by the thyroid gland. The diarrhea occurs from the increased intestinal motility that the excess thyroid hormone produces. This manifestation of a hyperthyroid state usually affects middle-aged people and is rarely seen in younger hyperthyroid patients. Many other diseases can result in diarrhea, but a complete discussion of all of them is beyond the scope of this book.

Summary

A diarrheal illness is unpleasant and potentially harmful to our health. It is important that adequate amounts of fluid be taken in during the time of any diarrheal illness to prevent the complication of severe dehydration. Each of us must find a regimen that will give us the best relief from the intestinal cramps and the need for frequent trips to the bathroom. For each this approach will be different. If any diarrheal illness lasts beyond five days, is associated with high continuous fevers, or is associated with blood within the diarrheal movements, a physician should be consulted immediately.

chapter ten

Hemorrhoids
and Anal Fissures

Hemorrhoids, or piles, as they are frequently called, are a frequent cause of discomfort and problems to millions of Americans. They are the most common GI tract illness that individuals have. Estimates reveal that probably 50 percent of all Americans have hemorrhoids either intermittently or permanently.[1] The problems that they cause vary considerably among individuals suffering from hemorrhoids.

Causes of Hemorroids

A hemorrhoid, or pile, is a dilated vein of the rectum and anal area. Hemorroids are the varicose veins of the rectum.[2] Humans are susceptible to the development of hemorrhoids for many reasons. The evolutionary development of man's upright position for walking causes increased pressure on the veins around the anus due to a gravity affect. Any situation in which the individual has to strain can result in an increased pressure within these veins. Therefore, straining to pass a constipated stool, coughing or sneezing, lifting heavy objects, and obesity are all common factors contributing to development of hemorrhoids.

Most pregnant women notice the presence of hemorrhoids before or after delivery of their baby. The straining at the time of delivery is probably the most important factor causing the hemorrhoids to develop. Once the hemorrhoids are present, they usually remain for the rest of one's life.

A common wives tale is that prolonged reading on the commode will cause hemorrhoids to develop. This position could predispose one to increased pressure within the perianal veins. Prolonged time on the commode might also indicate problems with a constipated stool, which would tend to increase the liklihood of hemorrhoidal development. It is possible that hemorrhoids could result after years of repetition of this reading habit. It should therefore be discouraged among individuals who practice it routinely.

The dilated rectal vein may be either internal or external in location. An external hemorrhoid develops in the veins that lie on the outside of the rectum. These may be felt as a lump adjacent to the rectal opening, which is known as the anus. An internal hemorrhoid cannot be felt during the personal hygiene of the rectal area. This type of hemorrhoid usually remains within the rectal canal and can only be detected during an examination of the rectum.

Some people with internal hemorrhoids will notice a prolapse or protrusion of the hemorrhoid through the anus during times of straining at defecation or with coughing or sneezing. In some the hemorrhoid will spontaneously return itself to its inner position within the rectum. In others the hemorrhoid will have to be manually returned to its position within the rectum. Finally, in some individuals the hemorrhoid becomes so stretched that it remains prolapsed through the anus at all times. A prolapsed hemorrhoid may

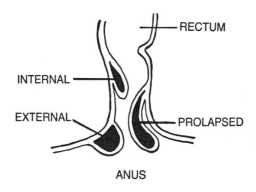

INTERNAL

EXTERNAL

RECTUM

PROLAPSED

ANUS

ILLUSTRATION 5. Hemorrhoids.

cause rectal seepage or a mucoid discharge to occur through the anus. This problem does not usually occur with hemorrhoids that remain in their internal position.

Symptoms of Hemorrhoids

What are the common symptoms of hemorrhoids or piles? The most common symptom that these dilated rectal veins produce is rectal bleeding. Bleeding associated with hemorrhoids is typically noticed on the tissue paper. Bright red blood will be noticed on the paper after wiping. Sometimes individuals with hemorrhoids will notice the streaking of blood on the sides of their stool. Rarely, there may be intense staining of the toilet bowl with blood. This occurs as the vein will sometimes rupture and blood will drip directly into the toilet bowl.

It is important that all individuals do not diagnose the cause of their rectal bleeding as due to hemorrhoids without proper medical advice. Persistent rectal bleeding at any age, but especially in people over forty years of age, is a mandatory reason to consult your physician. A proctoscopic examination will exclude a tumor of the lower large intestine and confirm that the bleeding is due to the presence of a hemorrhoid. However, I have seen many unfortunate individuals who have delayed their evaluation for up to six months, for they were sure their bleeding was due to hemorrhoids. Their diagnostic evaluation revealed a tumor as the cause of the rectal bleeding. Remember that any persistent rectal bleeding is a mandatory reason to see your physician.

Most individuals with hemorrhoids will notice some degree of rectal discomfort with a bowel movement. This rectal discomfort is worse with a constipated movement. Uncomplicated hemorrhoids do not cause intense pain in the anal area, usually. A thrombosed hemorrhoid may result in severe pain with walking, sitting, and at the time of defecation. A thrombosed hemorrhoid is one in which a blood clot has developed within the vein. The resultant situation is one of the most unpleasant that an individual can experience. Anyone who has experienced a thrombosed hemorrhoid knows the truth of the last sentence.

As previously mentioned, hemorrhoids may cause rectal itching or soiling of the undergarments. The itching and rectal soiling is due to the mucoid production of the rectum in response to the presence of the hemorrhoid. Needless to say, itching and further irritation of the rectal area only compound matters. The more we itch, the more irritation, the more itching and more soiling.

Treatment of Hemorrhoids

What is the most effective treatment of hemorrhoids? All sufferers of these rectal varicose veins must maintain regular bowel movements. Periods of prolonged constipation are to be avoided. Constipation necessitates the straining at the time of defecation. As previously stated, the straining can worsen the condition of the hemorrhoids. Bleeding from the hemorrhoids could also result from a constipated movement. The urge for a rectal evacuation should be answered quickly so that there is no increased pressure within the rectum.

A high-fiber diet and bulk laxatives have been of help to many individuals with hemorrhoids in maintaining bowel regularity. The method by which one can achieve bowel regularity with a high-fiber diet and bulk laxatives was discussed in Chapter 5. If you still have questions regarding a high-fiber diet or the use of bulk laxatives with a hemorrhoidal problem, your physician can help outline a program to help you.

What are the best general measures that can be taken to reduce the swelling of hemorrhoids? Warm sitz baths have long been recognized as an important part of the total approach to the care of hemorrhoids. Sufferers with hemorrhoids attest to the effectiveness of this technique in reducing the swelling and pain of hemorrhoids. This part of hemorrhoidal care is easily accomplished by taking a warm bath twice daily. If this warm bathtub routine is not effective, one should purchase from a pharmacy a regular sitz bath container to help reduce the swelling of hemorrhoids. Most individuals use only the warm water to reduce the swelling. Some individuals add various salt compounds to the bath water in an attempt to further reduce the swelling. Most physicians do not agree about the necessity of the addition of salts to the sitz bath.

There are many commercially available ointments that are designed for the purpose of reducing the swelling of hemorrhoidal tissue. People will state a difference in their response and the effectiveness of these various preparations. Try various different compounds and determine your own response. It may be necessary to consult your physician so that a prescription ointment can be given. Most ointments prescribed for hemorrhoidal problems contain various steroid compounds. These steroids are antiinflammatory agents that help reduce the swelling and inflammation of the hemorrhoidal tissue.

Prescription or nonprescription suppositories may also be used to help relieve your hemorrhoidal symptoms. The major difference between the two is the steroid content of the prescription suppositories.

The combination of the previously described remedies usually results in relief of the pain, swelling, and itching associated with active, inflamed hemorrhoids. Surgical procedures for the treatment of hemorrhoidal problems are limited to those individuals who fail to respond to the aforementioned maneuvers or have continued symptoms.

Before discussing the various surgical approaches to hemorrhoidal problems, it is important to remember that old external hemorrhoids don't fade away. These external hemorrhoids are replaced by skin tags that remain forever.[3] These skin tags do not cause symptoms but explain the redundant skin tissue that some sufferers of hemorrhoids notice. The majority of individuals with anal skin tags notice no problems with these tags in terms of their personal hygiene. These tags serve only as a remembrance of their former hemorrhoidal problems.

Surgical Treatment of Hemorrhoids

How are persistent and troublesome hemorrhoids treated? Some individuals will still require the surgical excision of hemorrhoids for relief of their symptoms. A hemorrhoidectomy, or the surgical removal of hemorrhoidal tissue, will require hospitalization, convalescent time, and the realization that this is a painful operation.[4] However, this is a highly effective method for treating recurrent hemorrhoidal problems. Many individuals with recurrent thrombosed hemorrhoids or persistent hemorrhoidal bleeding welcome the idea of hemorrhoid surgery. These individuals would rather have one painful operation than to experience the recurrence of their symptoms. I describe hemorrhoid surgery as painful because of the sensitivity of the area we are dealing with. However, other than the pain associated with their first postoperative bowel movement, the majority of individuals recover quickly from a hemorrhoidectomy.

Importantly, the recurrence of hemorrhoids after a hemorrhoid operation is low. This is in contrast to the relatively high incidence of recurrence after hemorrhoids have been removed using a rubber band technique. A rubber band is tied around the vein, which results in the vein being sloughed off after about seven days. This method appears to be simple and does not require hospitalization. The only drawback that I can see with this technique is the recurrence of the hemorrhoids after this procedure. Importantly, this procedure should be performed only by medically trained individuals and should not be tried by hemorrhoid sufferers themselves. There are serious potential complications that could result if this technique was performed by inexperienced hands.

Causes of Anal Fissures

Anal fissures are another common cause of anal itching and painful bowel movements. These fissures may predispose to bleeding with a bowel movement. The rectal bleeding has the same characteristics as the bleeding associated with hemorrhoids.

An anal fissure is a tear in the skin lining the anus. These anal skin tears are believed to result from the repetitive passage of large constipated stools. Most individuals with anal fissures will have a history of constipation that precedes the development of the fissures. A patient will occasionally develop an anal fissure after the passage of one large bowel movement.

An anal fissure may heal spontaneously or may persist and result in a chronic condition. Again, chronic anal fissure disease is most frequently seen in individuals with a history of chronic constipation. A persistent anal fissure can cause as many severe and recurrent symptoms as a chronic hemorrhoidal problem.

Some individuals with an anal fissure will experience the tearing or ripping burning pain with defecation. This pain results from the tearing of the lining of the rectum. This severe pain may last up to five or ten minutes after a bowel movement. The fear of experiencing this pain may

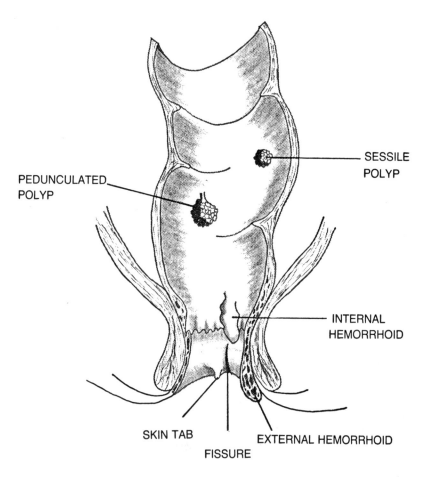

PEDUNCULATED POLYP

SESSILE POLYP

INTERNAL HEMORRHOID

SKIN TAB

FISSURE

EXTERNAL HEMORRHOID

ILLUSTRATION 6. Rectal Diseases.

cause these individuals to delay their bowel movement for days. This results in the passage of a larger, firmer stool. This makes the resultant delayed bowel movement very painful.

Treatment of Anal Fissures

An anal fissure can be easily diagnosed by an examination with a procto or anoscope. After the diagnosis is made, an anal fissure is treated identically to the general measures used in the therapy of hemorrhoids. The need for bowel regularity is mandatory. Sitz baths and topical ointments are important to reduce the swelling and inflammation. With the above program, most anal fissures will heal in seven to fourteen days.

The discouraging fact is that most anal fissures recur. This recurrence rate is related to the fact that after a couple of weeks of no rectal pain and regular bowel movements, sufferers become complacent in their treatment methods. Gradually the measures to prevent constipation are eliminated. Once constipation recurs, the likelihood of the recurrence of the anal fissure is high. Therefore, sufferers with anal fissures should dedicate themselves to the maintainance of a soft, regular bowel movement.

Anoscopy and Protoscopy as Diagnostic Tools

When discussing both hemorrhoidal and anal fissure problems, I have mentioned both *proctoscopy* and *anoscopy*. What do these terms mean? Anoscopy is the inspection of the anal area. Proctoscopy or proctosigmoidoscopy is the inspection of the rectum and lower portion of the large intestine, known as the sigmoid colon. These terms strike fear to the hearts of many. However, both of these diagnostic procedures should be relatively pain-free and be accomplished quickly. Certainly the apprehension that many individuals feel before having one of these diagnostic procedures contributes greatly to the need to have them performed properly. It is easy to say, but the most important thing to remember is the need to relax. Your relaxation will allow the physician to complete these simple diagnostic procedures more quickly.

How are these two diagnostic tests performed? Both will require an enema being given in the physician's office. After passage of the enema, the individual will be made to lie in one of a variety of positions. Most commonly, the patient lies on a procto table, which will first be elevated, then the head of the patient will be moved downward. If a procto table is unavailable, the patient may be asked to lie on his or her side, with the knees drawn up to the chest, or to assume a kneeling position with the hands on the examining table. Regardless of which position, remember the most important thing is to relax. First the physician will inspect the anus and the surrounding tissue. After this is accomplished, the doctor will examine the rectum with an examining finger. Many important facts may be learned by this digital examination. Not only can the rectum be evaluated for the presence of polyps or growth, but either the uterus or prostate gland can also be evaluated. Next the physician will pass a diagnostic tube through the anus into the rectum. Through this tube, the doctor can evaluate the anus, the rectum, and the lower portion of the large bowel. This instrument may give the patient the sensation of the need to have a bowel movement. Importantly, remember to relax; with proper relaxation, there are less bowel spasms and the diagnostic procedure is over more quickly. The average time for such an examination is only one to two minutes.

Why then do many individuals dislike having a procto? The reason is that as the diagnostic instrument advances upward into the rectum, the instrument encounters the normal curves within the large intestine. With passage around these curves, intestinal cramping can occur. These cramps are usually no more severe than those we have experienced with severe diarrhea. However, if we await these cramps with great intensity, we may make thngs worse. As I have repeated many times before, remember the need to relax; most of these diagnostic tests are completed within one to two minutes. There is good news for those individuals who cannot relax while having a procto. There are newer flexible instruments now available instead of the rigid proctosigmoidoscopes. These newer, flexible sigmoidoscopes will be discussed in Chapter 19.

Itching of the Perianal Area

Itching of the perianal area is a very common complaint among individuals consulting a digestive disease specialist or proctologist. Some individuals will have this bothersome complaint as a result of either an anal fissure or hemorrhoidal problems. However, the causes of pruritis ani, as itching of the perianal area is known, are multiple.[5] This itching can result as a consequence of a reaction to a new soap or laundry cleaner. The long-term usage of certain antibiotics may allow for the overgrowth of a certain fungus within this area. The combination of tight undergarments and obesity is a common reason why certain individuals will have rectal itching. Vigorous personal hygiene can result or perpetuate pruritis ani.

Pin worms are a common cause of anal itching in children. This is especially true if more than one child within the household is afflicted with pruritis ani. This cause of anal itching can be easily diagnosed with the tape test. The child is brought to the physician early in the morning before a bowel movement has occurred. The physician will then place a piece of scotch-like tape to the anal area. This tape will then be evaluated to see if the pin worms are found on the tape. It is important to remember that the child should not have a bowel movement before seeing the physician. The reason is that the pin worms migrate from the anus to the skin surrounding it. This occurs at nighttime. If the child has a movement, the act of personal hygiene may remove the pin worms and render the tape test invalid. Parents should consider this diagnosis when their children have persistent squirming due to rectal itching.

Treatment of Rectal Itching

Once the exact cause of the rectal itching has been determined, appropriate measures can be taken to correct it. An important first step is a change in the type of undergarments worn. The elimination of tight girdles or bedclothing has been found to be very helpful. A change in the technique of personal hygiene is also important. Less vigorous wiping is a necessity. The more wiping, the more irritation, the more itching. The use of Tucks pads, instead of toilet tissue, allows for proper cleansing but with a less bothersome effect. Tucks pads are a soft tissue containing glycerine and witch hazel. Some individuals use regular tissue paper gently and then apply either witch hazel or rubbing alcohol after its use. Both of these compounds help to dry the anal area. The application of petroleum jelly to the perianal area has been used by some suffering with nighttime pruritis ani. Importantly, if the measures just described do not result in the persistent resolution of this itching, it is sound medical advice to consult a physician.

Summary

The perianal area is the last part of our digestive tract. However, it is a frequent cause of problems for many Americans. Hemorrhoids and anal fissures are two reasons why the daily constitutional movement becomes an unpleasant and even feared experience. Pruritis ani is an unpleasant complaint that can cause loss of sleep and many nervous hours during the day.

chapter eleven

Living with
an Ileostomy
or Colostomy

Thousands of Americans are living full, productive lives with either an ileostomy or colostomy. Many of these individuals feared the name ileostomy or colostomy when they first heard it. They were afraid of the potential consequences that these surgically created bowel openings would have on their social or sexual lives. The vast majority of individuals with either an ileostomy or colostomy have noticed little or no change in their life styles.

What an Ileostomy Is

What is an ileostomy and what medical condition might necessitate the surgical formation of an ileostomy? An ileostomy results when the ileum, the end portion of the small intestine, is surgically brought out through the abdominal wall and is attached to the skin. An ileostomy is usually created when the surgical removal of the large intestine or colon is made necessary because of certain diseases. The digestive residue exits through the ileostomy opening, or stoma, into a bag which is fitted around the opening. This bag is known as an appliance.

An ileostomy may be performed as a temporary measure to rest a diseased large intestine afflicted by an inflammatory bowel disease state or a complication of diverticulitis. This procedure would remove the fecal stream away from the inflamed colon and allow for a quicker and more effective healing process. After healing of the large bowel has occurred, the ileostomy could be taken down and the normal digestive flow pattern reestablished. A permanent ileostomy is necessitated with the surgical removal of the colon. Inflammatory bowel disease of the colon is the most frequent reason why a permanent ileostomy would be created surgically.

Initially the patient with an ileostomy may notice a high output through the ileostomy opening. Frequently associated with this high ileostomy output will be a lot of gas production through the opening into the appliance. Gradually, as the small intestine adapts to the large bowel function, the ileostomy output will decrease in amount.

While hospitalized, the person will be instructed in the proper maintenance of their ostomy, skin care around the stoma, and procedures to deodorize the contents of the ileostomy bag. One of the patient's main concerns will be the proper care of the skin around the ileostomy opening. Meticulous care of this area will help prevent problems with skin infections and allow for the proper attachment of the appliance. Instructions will be given regarding dietary changes that can be useful in forming up the ileostomy output and in aiding the control of the odor of its contents.

In the past twenty years improved surgical techniques have reduced the problems that were formerly associated with some ileostomies. Most of the problems were related to the opening, or stoma, of the ileostomy. In the past many ileostomy openings had become narrowed and did not function properly. Today an ileostomy may still require surgical revision but less frequently than in the past.

Patients with an ileostomy are encouraged to join local and national ileostomy societies. At these meetings the individual will receive information about common problems relating to ileostomy care and ileostomy functioning. They are able to discuss their feelings regarding sexual relationships with an ileostomy or how to overcome the feeling of body embarrassment that some individuals with an ileostomy have. These ileostomy societies are one reason for the social and economic success of many individuals with an ileostomy.

The United Ostomy Association, 111 Wilshire Blvd., Los Angeles, California, is one national group that has been of assistance to ileostomy patients. I encourage all of my patients with an ileostomy to join either a local or national group because of the assistance given in regard to the social and psychological aspects of living with an ileostomy.

Is there a new type of bagless ileostomy? Recently, an internal or continent ileostomy has been developed.[1] This type of ileostomy has the end portion of the small intestine formed into a pouch that lies beneath the skin. This pouch takes the place of the bag or appliance. A tube is inserted through a surgically created hole in the skin to drain the contents. Early studies performed on individuals with this type of ileostomy reveal encouraging results.[2] This internal ileostomy is especially suitable for adolescents and young adults because it eliminates many of the concerns about potential social and sexual problems. It also reduces the concerns about unpleasant bag odors and skin irritation.

The creation of a continent ileostomy can either be done at the time of the first operation or be performed after an external ileostomy has already been created. Which type of ileostomy is formed will depend upon the surgeon involved, the disease for which the ileostomy is created, and the individual's understanding of the care and potential problems with both types of ileostomies.

What a Colostomy Is

What is a colostomy, and is a colostomy performed for different medical reasons than an ileostomy? A colostomy results from the surgical creation of an opening of the large bowel through the abdominal wall onto the skin. As with ileostomies, colostomies may be permanent or temporary. A temporary colostomy is usually performed to divert the digestive waste stream from an area of inflammation within the lower segment of the large intestine. This allows that area to be freed of contamination and facilitates healing. Colonic abscesses and fistulas may be treated in this way.

Most permanent colostomies are performed on patients with cancer of the colon or female organs that have resulted in blockage of the large bowel. In some of these cases the tumor is unable to be surgically removed. The colostomy allows for proper elimination of the digestive tract residue while the cancer is treated with drugs and radiation treatments. In certain cases the tumor could be surgically removed, but there is insufficient length of the large intestine to allow for a proper reconnection. These individuals can be surgically cured of their cancer but have a permanent colostomy.

It is easily seen why individuals' fear of a colostomy results not only from the colostomy itself, but also from the reason why the colostomy had to be formed. In discussions with patients known to have a large bowel tumor, they frequently ask what the chances are that they will require a colostomy. I try to explain the reasons why a colostomy may be necessary and to explain how people function actively with a colostomy. Most of these individuals have persistent fear of a colostomy despite this type of discussion. This fear is mainly related to the realization that they have a cancer. The colostomy will be an outward sign of this fact to them and their family.

Most individuals with a colostomy, especially those surgically cured of a cancer that necessitated the colostomy, live productive lives after adapting to their stoma. This requires overcoming the psychological presence of the colostomy and then learning to care for it. Conversations with other colostomy patients are helpful in assisting these patients. These discussions allow for the hashing over of psychological concerns and the best way to manage a colostomy. Patients with a colostomy will use their appliances in different ways to handle the digestive tract waste. Some individuals will prefer to wear the colostomy appliance at all times and allow the output to enter it. Other people would prefer to develop a schedule of irrigating or flushing out their colon. This daily routine removes the digestive waste and enables these individuals to wear only a gauze pad instead of the somewhat bulky appliance. Initially during irrigation training the apparatus may be required to prevent accidental spillage. After the bowel is trained, many individuals are able to wear only a gauze pad.

Patients with either an ileostomy or colostomy will learn what dietary changes are needed to maintain proper functioning of their stomas. They learn what foods will result in an increased ostomy output, gas production, and malodorousness to the ostomy output. By eliminating these foods, these problems can be avoided.

Rarely, patients with an ostomy will notice bleeding through the stoma. This stoma bleeding is usually associated with heavy lifting or strenuous exercise. This bleeding is usually small in amount and quickly stops. These physical activities result in an increased pressure within the abdominal cavity. This increased pressure is transmitted to the thin wall veins within the ostomy. These vessels may rupture, and bleeding through the stoma results. If this occurrence is noted, these activities should be avoided. If bleeding occurs regularly and is not related to physical activity, the patient should consult a physician immediately. This particular situation requires medical evaluation to determine the cause of the bleeding.

An important role is played by the family and loved ones of individuals with either an ileostomy or colostomy. They must lend support and understanding to the ostomy patient. They should encourage active discussions about any facet of life that may cause psychological or social embarrassment to the ostomy patient. In this way ostomy patients can avoid situations in which they would be uncomfortable.

Summary

The stigma presently attached to an ileostomy or colostomy must be corrected by a better understanding of these surgically created bowel openings. These ostomies are formed because of certain digestive diseases. The presence of an ostomy does not prohibit an individual from living an active, productive life. Patience and understanding by the patients and their families are required to enable the proper care of the ostomy and to overcome any possible psychological acceptance problems. Local and national ostomy clubs are available and very helpful in this regard.

chapter twelve
Ulcerative Colitis

Ulcerative colitis is characterized by inflammation of the lining of the large bowel or colon. This digestive disease represents a true colitis or inflamed colon with ulcerations found in the mucosa or lining of the large bowel. It is a chronic disease characterized by periods of exacerbations and remissions. The natural history is one of flare-ups with active symptoms at times, and other times with no active symptoms. The cause of this chronic digestive disease remains unknown, despite extensive medical research. This form of colitis is associated with a high rate of disability because of its severity and chronicity.

Mucosal ulcerative colitis, as this disease is known in the medical literature, is distinct from the irritable bowel syndrome or tension-related colitis. The latter digestive disease is not an inflammation of the colon but results from the abnormal motility of the bowel. Unfortunately individuals with ulcerative colitis merit this term with the chronic inflammatory condition of their large intestine. Fortunately the majority of Americans stating that they have colitis actually have an irritable bowel syndrome.

Ulcerative colitis is a disease that shows no preferences. Any American may be afflicted with this disease. It knows no barriers for sex, age, or race. Earlier medical reports revealed a tendency for ulcerative colitis to occur more commonly in the higher socioeconomic classes, in individuals with a higher level of education, and in whites as compared with nonwhites. More recent studies confirm the higher incidence in whites but fail to demonstrate a difference relating to the socioeconomic or educational status of the individual. Today ulcerative colitis is recognized in both rural and urban environments. Initial medical data seemed to indicate a higher frequency of the disease within an urban setting.

Ulcerative colitis is recognized most frequently in the twenty- to forty-year age group. It rarely occurs in individuals younger than twenty years of age but it can affect people over the age of fifty-five. Recent evidence seems to indicate that this digestive disease can affect the fifty- to seventy-year-old age group with the same severity as the younger individuals. There is no readily available explanation for the distinct separate occurrence rates within these two age groups. It is important to remember that this inflammatory bowel disease can affect anyone at any age. Medical studies demonstrate only the tendency or prevalence for the disease to occur.

Causes of Ulcerative Colitis

The cause of ulcerative colitis remains unknown.[1] An infectious etiology has not been demonstrated. No virus, bacteria, or parasite has been shown to predictably cause ulcerative colitis. These infectious agents are known reasons that certain individuals develop an episode of acute colitis. These infectious inflammations of the colon respond to antibiotic therapy and are rarely recurring. Genetic factors have been studied and do not appear to have an important role in the causation of ulcerative colitis. However, ulcerative colitis does occur more commonly in certain families.[2] Usually the disease is not seen in children of an affected individual, but rather the aunts, uncles or cousins of that person may develop ulcerative colitis. Therefore, a genetic predisposition exists for the development of mucosal colitis. The exact hereditary factors responsible for this are not known. Indeed, it may be necessary that a combination of genetic factors and an exposure to something in our environment is required for the causation of mucosal ulcerative colitis.[3]

Though the exact cause of ulcerative colitis remains to be defined, various reasons exist why flare-ups of activity of this disease occur. People with ulcerative colitis develop viral and bacterial infections of their digestive tracts, as we all can. However, these infections are more troublesome and resolve more slowly in those individuals. Indeed, a viral illness such as the common cold could result in active symptoms in a patient with ulcerative colitis. Periods of increased emotional stress or tension have been associated with exacerbations of symptoms in certain individuals with ulcerative colitis.

Ulcerative colitis is a disease that is variable in its course and severity.[4] In most individuals the disease is characterized by periods of active symptoms followed by asymptomatic time periods. This intermittent and recurrent form of ulcerative colitis is most commonly observed. Less commonly, an individual will have continuous symptoms for a prolonged time period. Some may have symptoms for years without relief. Rarely, an individual will have only one attack of documented ulcerative colitis and never experience further problems.

Symptoms of Active Ulcerative Colitis

What are the symptoms observed in individuals with active ulcerative colitis? The majority of sufferers will notice the onset of diarrhea, rectal bleeding with bowel movements, crampy abdominal pain, and some amount of weight loss.

The diarrhea and the belly cramps will start suddenly. Most individuals can easily remember the date of the onset of these symptoms. The diarrhea is associated with extreme urgency, and soiling accidents are not uncommon. The need for the passage of loose bowel movements may occur during the sleeping hours and awaken the person many times during the night. The number of movements is variable, but the average with a flare-up can approach ten to twenty times daily. Commonly the severity of the intestinal cramps is relieved with a diarrheal episode.

A bloody bowel movement is characteristic of ulcerative colitis. Not uncommonly an individual may have rectal urgency and pass only bloody mucoid material. The amount of blood passed varies considerably among ulcerative colitics but is usually sufficient to color the commode water red. At the time the bloody diarrhea is noticed, the individual may feel feverish, weak, and tired. His or her appetite decreases, and weight loss of variable amounts is commonly seen.

Generally those people having more severe symptoms will have more intense inflammation of the lining of their colons.[5] The amount of colon involved with inflammation will vary among individuals with ulcerative colitis. In most the entire large bowel will be inflamed, while in others only segments of the lower colon will be diseased. The greater the amount of colon involvement, the more severe the symptoms usually. Therefore, the severity of symptoms is a good indicator of the length of colon involved and the degree of inflammation present.

People with the severe form of ulcerative colitis are sicker, respond less favorably to treatment, and require more frequent hospitalizations.[6] These individuals have a higher rate of complications and a higher death rate than those afflicted with a milder form of this disease. If individuals who have the severe form of ulcerative colitis survive the first three years, their complication and death rates return to that of individuals with the milder form of the disease.

Ulcerative colitis is a digestive disease that deserves our respect. The severity of this illness and its complications make it important that individuals with ulcerative colitis follow their physicians' orders faithfully. Medications should be taken as prescribed, and those individuals should notify their physician when recurrent symptoms occur.

Diagnosis and Treatment of Ulcerative Colitis

The diagnosis of ulcerative colitis can usually be established quite easily. A proctoscopic or proctosigmoidoscopic examination will give the physician valuable information. This diagnostic test has been previously described in Chapter 10. This examination allows the physician to visually inspect the lining of the large bowel and rectum and take tissue samples or biopsy specimens for evaluation under the microscope. During this short procedure stool specimens can also be obtained for analysis. This evaluation will exclude a bacterial or parasitic cause of the inflammation. If the procto exam suggests the diagnosis of ulcerative colitis, the stool analysis excludes an infectious cause, and the tissue samples confirm the characteristics of this disease, a diagnosis has been made.

The extent of inflammation within the colon must now be determined. The proctoscopic examination evaluates only the lower portion of the colon, known as the rectosigmoid area. A barium X-ray test must be performed to determine what extent of the remaining large bowel is involved with this disease. This examination will probably be performed after the diarrhea and the rectal bleeding have lessened with treatment. The treatment of ulcerative colitis will depend upon the amount of colon involvement, the severity of the symptoms, and the individual's drug allergy history.[7] A sulfa drug and steroid compounds remain the mainstay of treatment of this disease. Both medications have an effect of decreasing inflammation within the large intestine. This antiinflammatory effect is accomplished by a different mechanism with each drug.

The sulfa drug is known as sulfasalazine. This specific sulfa drug is not an antibiotic. It works differently from other sulfa medications. It is not designed to treat bladder or kidney infections. Sulfasalazine is used to reduce the inflammation within the colon, associated with ulcerative colitis. Many studies attest to its effectiveness in this regard. There is evidence to suggest that this drug can also prevent recurrences or flare-ups from developing in individuals with ulcerative colitis.[8]

Unfortunately many individuals who would benefit from this sulfa drug cannot take this medication because of their allergy to sulfa medications. Most commonly those individuals will have noticed a skin rash or hives with prior sulfa usage. Other people might have experienced nausea or vomiting while taking sulfa medications. It is important that you mention your drug allergy history to your physician. It is possible that some people may be able to tolerate sulfasalazine. Newer preparations of this medication have enabled certain individuals to tolerate the drug despite their allergic history. Other sufferers with ulcerative colitis have been desensitized to this drug and are able to tolerate the medication in full dosage strength. There are various steroid or cortisone preparations that can be used in the treatment of ulcerative colitis.[9] The ability of this type of medication to reduce inflammation has resulted in its usage in many disease states. Steroid creams are utilized for various skin rashes, and some steroid preparations are used to treat certain forms of arthritis. When the inflammation with ulcerative colitis is limited to the lower rectosigmoid colon, steroid-containing enemas, foam preparation, or suppositories can be used. The rectal administration of these compounds enables a direct effect on the inflamed lining of the colon. If the colitis is severe or involves the total colon, the medication may have to be given orally.

This powerful antiinflammatory medicine merits our respect when taken orally or systemically in high dosages. During such therapy the adrenal glands decrease their production of steroid hormones. Therefore, the only source of these important hormones are those taken daily. If the individual could not take the medication because of nausea or vomiting, the body would be without a supply of vital metabolism-controlling substance. If this situation occurs, that person should contact his or her physician immediately. If one is unable to do so, proceed directly to an emergency room. For the same reason, high-dose steroid medication should never be stopped indiscriminately without a physician's recommendation. This form of treatment demands your respect and understanding of its usage.

Most of the severe cases of ulcerative colitis will respond to systemic steroid treatment. The length of time required to take this type of medication will vary, dependent upon the severity of the inflammation and the extent of disease within the colon. Physicians use steroid-containing drugs to maximize the healing process in the shortest amount of time.

Ulcerative colitis is one digestive disease that affects the health of those afflicted with it in two important ways. First I have mentioned the chronic and recurrent nature of the inflammation within the colon. Each acute episode will vary in severity and in the ability to produce a healing of the acute inflammation. Secondly there is medical data to suggest that ulcerative colitis is a precancerous condition.[10] The evidence seems to indicate that people with ulcerative colitis have an increased risk for the development of cancer of the colon when compared with healthy individuals of the same age group. The length of time one has ulcerative colitis and the amount of colon involved are important factors regarding the risk of cancer. Individuals with the colitis limited to the rectosigmoid colon, or the lower portion of the large bowel, are not at an increased risk for the development of cancer of the colon.

Individuals with total colon involvement with ulcerative colitis of longer than ten years duration must be followed closely. The colitis may not have been active for a few years, but these individuals need to have their colons checked for early signs of cancer.[11] If any abnormalities are found, your physician will probably recommend the removal of the chronically inflamed colon. This surgery could prevent cancer from developing.

Surgical Treatment of Ulcerative Colitis

What is the surgical treatment of ulcerative colitis? It is important to remember that ulcerative colitis involves only the large bowel and not the small intestine. Therefore, surgical removal of the entire colon, or colectomy, with the formation of an ileostomy, is curative of this disease. An ileostomy is an opening of the end of the small intestine on the abdominal wall.

When is surgery usually recommended to patients having ulcerative colitis? The surgical removal of the colon may be necessary in cases of severe colitis that fail to respond to intense medical therapy.[12] Certain individuals with severe ulcerative colitis will need emergency surgery for the condition known as a toxic megacolon.[13] The removal of the severely inflamed colon, with this complication of ulcerative colitis, may be lifesaving. A toxic megacolon occurs when the diseased colon stops functioning properly, swells or dilates and may perforate, or pops spontaneously. The term *toxic* indicates the severity and seriousness of this condition. Rarely, a colectomy must be performed to stop the uncontrolled bleeding from a colon inflamed with ulcerative colitis. Finally the elective removal of the colon may be performed because of the increased cancer risk in certain individuals with ulcerative colitis.

Various types of ileostomies, including the pouch or Koch ileostomy, have been reviewed in Chapter 11. Most individuals having a colectomy with an ileostomy notice improvement in their sense of health after surgery. Weight gain and increased vitality and sense of well-being are commonly noticed after the surgical removal of the inflamed large intestine. Certainly the presence of an ileostomy does not affect the activities of most individuals.

Summary

Ulcerative colitis is a chronic digestive disease that adversely affects the normal life style of those affected with it. Not only are the physical consequences of this inflammatory condition of the colon important; also, the psychological impact of this disease is varied and potentially severe. Because of the physical limitations that result from this disease, feelings of inadequacy regarding income generation, sexual relationships, and family participation may develop. The chronic severe nature of this illness has a tendency to result in depression. Those unfortunate individuals with ulcerative colitis need support and understanding from their families and loved ones. Once the mental strain of the acute attack of colitis has been resolved, the concern of the cancer risk becomes evident. It is important to stress open relationships and discussion about such feelings between patients and physicians or family members. In this manner potentially severe psychological consequences could be averted.

chapter thirteen
Crohn's Disease

Crohn's disease is a chronic inflammation of the digestive tract. This disease can affect any part of the digestive system, from the mouth to the perianal area. Crohn's disease is characterized by an inflammation that involves all the layers of the gut wall. Besides this transmural, or total wall, involvement a unique type of inflammation known as granuloma is commonly found in the digestive tract of individuals suffering with Crohn's disease. Unlike ulcerative colitis, this digestive illness frequently results in fistulae, or connections, between the involved digestive tract and other body structures. The medical treatment of Crohn's disease is similar to that for ulcerative colitis. However, unlike ulcerative colitis, surgery does not guarantee a cure with this disease. Crohn's disease can recur in another part of the digestive tract after surgery.

This digestive disease was formerly known as *regional enteritis.*[1] This term describes the involvement of the small intestine and the tendency of this illness to be patchy in its distribution. The inflammation has the tendency to be nonuniform in nature or have normal intestine amid surrounding areas of inflammation. Hence, the regional aspect of the descriptive medical name. Dr. Isadore Crohn and his associates wrote many important papers on regional enteritis in the 1930s. Today this disease bears his name as a tribute to his work.[2]

Crohn's disease most commonly affects the small intestine or colon. Less commonly the stomach and duodenum are involved with this illness. Rarely the esophagus is detected to have Crohn's disease. Commonly both the end portion of the small intestine, known as the ileum, and the large bowel or colon are found involved with this disease. *Granulomatous enterocolitis,* or granulomatous inflammation of the small and large intestine, is the medical term used to describe this particular involvement with Crohn's disease.

As with ulcerative colitis, the cause or etiology of Crohn's disease remains unknown.[3] What is known is that the incidence or the recognition of new cases of Crohn's disease is increasing yearly.[4] Not only are physicians more aware of this illness, but also medical data would support the fact that more individuals are developing Crohn's disease. The reason for this increased incidence, especially in industrialized Northern Hemisphere countries, is presently being evaluated.

The characteristic involvement of all the layers of the digestive tract results in many important consequences.[5] The mucosa or lining of the gut is involved with an ulcerative inflammation that is distinct from ulcerative colitis. These ulcerations can result in the loss of blood, protein, and fluids through the inflamed lining layer. Anemia, weight loss, or malnutrition and dehydration can be resultant effects. The inflammatory reaction in the muscle and coating or serosal layer of the digestive tract results in the thickening and scarring of the bowel. Narrowings or strictures of the involved segment could lead to obstruction or blockage of the digestive tract.

The inflammation of the outer two layers in the intestine can result in connections being established between the diseased bowel and other organs such as the urinary bladder, female organs, other areas of the digestive tract, and the skin. The connections are known as fistulas. Fistulas frequently complicate Crohn's disease when it involves the end portion of the small intestine alone, or in conjunction with the colon or large intestine. These connections cause much of the disability associated with Crohn's disease and may necessitate an operation for their resolution.

Individuals with Crohn's disease will have different symptoms dependent upon what section of the digestive tract is involved with the inflammation. An important feature of this illness is the variable presentation in different individuals having the same digestive organ involvement. What are some of the common symptoms that people with Crohn's disease have?

Symptoms of Crohn's Disease

Individuals with Crohn's disease of the small intestine usually have diarrhea or loose, frequent bowel movements. The diarrhea may or may not contain visible blood. Crampy abdominal pains are frequently associated with the loose movements. Weight loss, variable degrees of malnutrition, and anemia are commonly observed in these individuals. Malaise and fatigability are noticed secondary to the blood loss, anemia, or malnutrition. In addition, some individuals will demonstrate evidence of vitamin deficiencies. The malnutrition, weight loss, and lack of certain vitamins result from the inflamed small intestine being unable to absorb ingested food properly.

Some people with small intestinal Crohn's disease will develop obstruction of the intestinal flow as a result of the fibrous scarring. These individuals usually experience severe cramping, belly pains, and vomiting after eating meals. The symptoms may not occur with liquids or soft foods. Because these unfortunate individuals wish to prevent such symptoms from occurring, they eat less, and further weight loss and malnutrition occurs.

Individuals with granulomatous colitis, or Crohn's disease of the colon, have symptoms similar to those experienced by people with ulcerative colitis. Bloody diarrhea is the most frequent complaint. Weight loss and various degrees of malnutrition result from the body utilizing the caloric and protein intake in an attempt to heal this chronic inflammation of the colon. Crohn's colitis is associated with the same complications as ulcerative colitis. Toxic megacolon, severe bleeding or hemorrhage from the inflamed colon, fistulas, and cancer of the colon can occur as complications of granulomatous colitis.[6]

There appears to be a slight increased risk of developing cancer of the colon after having long-standing severe Crohn's colitis.[7] The magnitude of this potential complication is small when compared with that of patients with severe ulcerative colitis of ten years duration. Digestive disease specialists are concerned about this potential complication, especially with the increased recognition of more new cases of Crohn's disease.

The natural history of Crohn's disease is similar to that of ulcerative colitis. There are periods of exacerbations or increased activity of the disease, followed by remissions or improvements in the amount of inflammation. Some important differences exist between ulcerative colitis and Crohn's disease. Ulcerative colitis involves only the colon, while Crohn's disease can affect any part of the digestive tract. Secondly surgical removal of a colon involved with ulcerative colitis is curative of the disease. Unfortunately Crohn's disease has a significant recurrence rate after surgery.[8] The disease tends to occur proximal, or in a part of the digestive tract closer to the mouth than the section surgically removed. Therefore, if the colon was removed for a complication of Crohn's disease, the disease might recur in the small intestine. If the end portion of the small bowel was removed, the recurrence of the disease might be in the upper or middle portion of the small intestine. This observed phenomenon is known as the proximal rule of recurrence of Crohn's disease.

The recurrence rate of Crohn's disease makes physicians more vigorous in their medical treatment of this disease. Unfortunately the chronic progressive nature of this illness and its many complications require that surgery be performed. Dr. Richard Farmer of the Cleveland Clinic, a world-recognized authority on Crohn's disease, has demonstrated that a second surgical operation will be needed in approximately 40 percent of the patients within fifteen years of their first operation for Crohn's disease.[9]

The medical treatment of Crohn's disease is directed at the reduction of the inflammation within the diseased bowel segment. Steroid medications and the sulfa drug, sulfasalazine, are the mainstays in its treatment. The reason for the usage of these drugs and their potential side effects were discussed in Chapter 12. Medical data has shown that the sulfa drug is more effective in colon disease and that the steroid medications are more effective in the treatment of Crohn's disease of the small bowel.[10]

Crohn's disease involving the small intestine and colon present many serious considerations for both the patient and the physician. Evidence shows that this combined involvement is associated with the highest complication rate, the greatest need for surgery, and a higher recurrence rate after surgery. The small intestinal disease requires the usage of long-term high-dose steroid medication for its treatment. Therefore, therapy for this form of the disease has a higher incidence of complications.

Surgery will be required in some patients with Crohn's disease. This may be necessary for either the complications of the original disease or to treat a recurrence that is uncontrolled by medical management. A few unfortunate individuals with Crohn's disease will require multiple operations to control their disease activity. In a few of these individuals the remaining normal digestive tract will be

inadequate to perform its function. There is not enough intestine to digest and absorb ingested food. How will these individuals eat and receive their required nutrition?

Some of these people with a short bowel will be able
to ingest special food preparations. These elemental diets, as
they are known, contain carbohydrates, protein, fats, vitamins, and minerals in a predigested and readily absorbable
form. This type of diet was originally used on the space
flights because of its complete nutritional formula and low
residue component. Some people will not be able to tolerate
these preparations and require permanent intravenous, or
in-the-vein, feedings for their nutrition. This form of nutrition is known as total parenteral nutrition, or
hyperalimentation. A large bore flexible catheter is placed
within a large vein in the neck or shoulder area. Intravenous
solutions are infused through this I.V. as the individual
sleeps at night. These solutions provide all their nutritional
requirements. By using either technique, the oral or intravenous route, most of these unfortunate individuals are able to
maintain their weight and proper nutritional status. Some
have even been able to return to work or complete their educational studies.

Summary

Crohn's disease is a chronic digestive illness that has a great
socioeconomic impact on those afflicted by it. Unfortunately
this disease seems to be increasing in its recognition and occurrence. The therapy of this chronic illness has been improved, but many individuals still languish in its effects.
Crohn's disease has many associated complications that may
require surgery. It is hoped that the cause of this disease will
be identified in the future so that measures can be taken to
prevent its occurrence.

chapter fourteen

Diseases of the Gallbladder

More than 20 million Americans suffer with gallbladder disease. The majority of these people will have gallstones as the source of their problem. Diseases of this digestive organ are so common that gallbladder surgery has become one of the most common elective operations being performed in America.[1] Why people develop gallstones, which individuals may require gallbladder surgery, and the newer nonsurgical techniques of gallstone therapy will be discussed in this chapter.

What purpose does the gallbladder normally serve? The gallbladder is a reservoir for the storage of bile, which is produced and secreted by the liver. Bile has an important function in the digestion of fatty foods. Fatty foods, while in the stomach and duodenum, stimulate a hormone to be secreted into the blood. This hormone, known as cholecystokinin, causes the gallbladder to contract and pro-pel the bile downward into the bile ducts and the small intes-tine. Once in the small bowel, the bile interacts with the in-gested fats to help in their digestive process. The active component of the bile is known as bile acids.

There are tubes or bile ducts that convey the bile from the liver to the gallbladder. The main bile duct is known as the common bile duct. The gallbladder drains into this duct. The common bile duct empties into the small intes-tine through an opening known as the papilla of Vater. The pancreas duct drains through the same opening as the com-mon bile duct. The close relationship of these two ducts will be discussed later in connection with the causes of acute in-flammation within the pancreas by gallstones passing down the common bile duct.

Gallbladder disease is more frequent in females than in males. Evidence would suggest that the female hormones make the bile more susceptible to the formation of gall-stones. Women who have been pregnant one or more times have a higher incidence of gallstone-related gallbladder dis-ease than women who have never been pregnant. Women who have taken birth control pills for a long time and have never been pregnant have a high incidence of gallstone-related gallbladder disease. These two observations lend sup-port to the concept that the female hormones make the bile more susceptible to gallstone formation and to a greater need for gallbladder surgery.[2]

There is a medical expression about gallbladder dis-ease that reads: "female, forty, fat, flatulence and fatty food intolerance."[3] This easily memorized statement has been part of medical school training for years. It summarizes many of the facts that are related to gallbladder disease. As previously mentioned, females are more likely to have gallbladder disease than men. Individuals usually notice the onset of symptoms around the age of forty. Recently younger and younger women are being diagnosed with gallbladder disease. The role that the "pill" has played in causing the earlier onset of symptomatic gallbladder disease is an interesting source of speculation. The fat component of

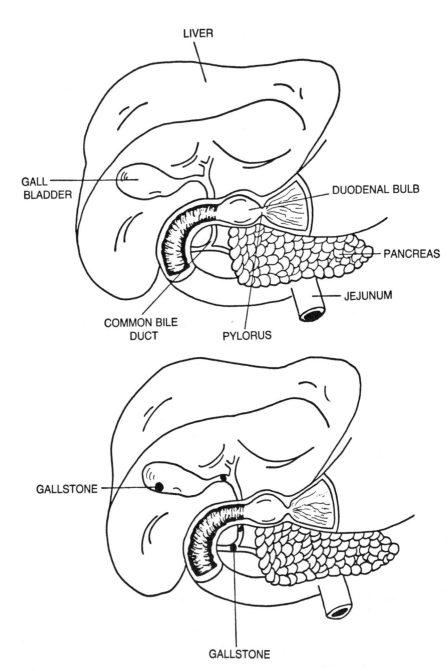

ILLUSTRATION 7. Liver, Gallbladder, and Pancreas.

this expression relates to a frequently observed association of gallbladder disease with overweight, middle aged females. Some individuals having an abnormal functioning or diseased gallbladder will notice an intolerance to fatty foods. If these individuals eat fatty foods, they frequently notice the onset of unpleasant symptoms. These symptoms are known as flatulent dyspepsia. Belching, flatulence, abdominal bloating, and abdominal discomfort can occur after dietary indiscretion. Not all individuals with gallbladder disease will be intolerant of fatty foods. More importantly, not all individuals with fatty food intolerance will have gallbladder disease. Many individuals with an irritable bowel will notice these symptoms after eating fatty foods. These symptoms result from the influence of the released cholecystokinin hormone increasing the number and severity of bowel spasms. This fact may cause confusion for both the patient and physician.

How Gallstones Are Formed

What is a gallstone? Is there more than one type of gallstone? How does a gallstone cause gallbladder or biliary pain? A gallstone is like a kidney stone in many aspects. A stone is formed when the concentration of certain substances within the bile or urine becomes so high that it settles or precipitates out. With gallstones, the focus for the formation is cholesterol crystals. Most gallstones contain some calcium bilirubinate. Individuals with a congenital hemolytic anemia, such as sickle-cell anemia or Cooley's anemia, will have a greater concentration of calcium bilirubinate in their gallstones. The gallstones of a hematologic origin are usually darker in color than normal gallstones. The calcium content allows for the gallstone to be seen with an X-ray. A gallstone is therefore a combination of cholesterol crystals, calcium, and bilirubinate deposits. Gallstones are known medically by the term *cholelithiasis*.

Like a kidney stone, a gallstone can cause an individual great pain and the need for admission to the hospital.

Gallstones are associated with most diseases of the gallbladder or bile ducts. These diseases result when the gallstone blocks the exit from the gallbladder to the main bile duct or when the stone passes into the common bile duct and becomes lodged there. A stone blocking any tubular structure causes severe colicky pain. This duct could be either the main bile duct or the ureter, which connects the kidney and urinary bladder.

Most individuals with gallstones experience episodic attacks of pain in the right side of their upper abdomen. This pain may vary in its intensity in a cyclic nature, so it is known as a colicky pain. While individuals are experiencing biliary colic, they cannot sit still and are very restless. The pain seems to radiate or move beneath the right shoulder blade in about half of the individuals. This pain could result from either a gallstone blocking the exit of the gallbladder or passing into the main bile duct. Biliary colic compares in its severity to the passage of a kidney stone.

An acute inflammation of the gallbladder, known as acute cholecystitis, can occur in any patient with gallbladder disease. The acute inflammation is felt to result from the blockage of bile outflow from the gallbladder.[4] In the majority of cases, gallstones are believed responsible for this blockage. However, in some cases of acute cholecystitis, spasms of the outflow duct from the gallbladder are felt to cause the blockage. Why and how does the obstruction of bile outflow from the gallbladder result in acute cholecystitis?

Causes of Acute Cholecystitis

This situation is somewhat analogous to blowing up a balloon. As the balloon becomes bigger, its walls become thinner and tense. When the bile outflow is blocked, the walls of the gallbladder become taut as it enlarges. This increased pressure within the walls of the gallbladder reduces the blood flow within them. This combination of the bile outflow blockage and the decreased blood flow within the gallbladder predisposes the individual to bacterial infection.[5] Acute cholecystitis results.

The majority of individuals having acute cholecystitis have a history of at least one attack of biliary colic pain. This data lends support to the theory that gallstones are the most common cause of bile outflow obstruction of the gallbladder. It is not known why gallstones that have been present in the gallbladder for some time suddenly cause problems. It is the rare person who develops an acute attack of cholecystitis after eating a fatty meal. Therefore, it is not likely that the contracting gallbladder forces the stones into the outflow or exit duct and causes the blockage.

Individuals experiencing an episode of acute cholecystitis will notice the onset of pain similar to biliary colic pain that has been described. In addition, the person feels ill, and may have a fever and associated nausea and vomiting. Jaundice, the yellowish discoloration of the skin and eyes, does not usually occur with acute gallbladder inflammation unless a gallstone has passed into the common bile duct and lodged there. Anyone experiencing these symptoms should notify a physician immediately.

If a gallstone becomes lodged in the main bile duct and blocks the bile outflow, an individual will experience the symptoms just described. Besides fever, they may have a teeth-rattling, shaking chill. Commonly there is the observed yellowish hue to the whites of the eye and the skin. This jaundice results from the backing up of bile pigment into the bloodstream. This pigment is known as bilirubin. The clearance of the bilirubin in the blood by the kidneys causes the urine to have a dark coke-like color. The failure of the bile and this pigment to pass into the small intestine results in the bowel movements being a light tan color.

A blockage of the common bile duct can cause an inflammation of the bile. This bacterial infection is known as a cholangitis. This type of infection is commonly associated with the bacteria entering the bloodstream so that sepsis, or blood poisoning, exists. The shaking chill may be a sign of this infection. Gallstone-related bile duct infection, or cholangitis, is a medical emergency with potentially serious complications. If you have the symptoms just described seek medical attention promptly.

Gallbladder disease can be diagnosed by the recognition of typical clinical symptoms and different X-ray studies of the gallbladder. The symptoms of gallbladder disease have been previously discussed. How are gallbladder X-rays done, and what do they tell your doctor about the gallbladder's function? The oral cholecystogram, the commonly used X-ray study of the gallbladder, is performed by having an individual take two to four tablets the evening before the examination. These tablets contain X-ray dye, which is taken up by the liver and excreted into the bile. The bile is stored overnight in the gallbladder. In the morning an X-ray is taken of the abdomen, which demonstrates the gallbladder outlined by the dye within it.

If an individual has chronic gallbladder disease or an acutely inflamed gallbladder, the X-ray will not demonstrate this digestive organ. This is referred to as a nonvisualized gallbladder examination. It results from the inability of the gallbladder to concentrate the X-ray dye to a degree that it can be visualized. If a patient has gallstones, they would be visualized in the dye-filled gallbladder.

The limitations of the oral cholecystogram study are evident in some cases of patients in whom the existence of gallstones has been surgically proven, but in whom no gallstones were seen with this X-ray technique. Also, individuals with symptoms indicative of chronic gallbladder disease may have a normal oral cholecystogram. However, when surgery is performed because of their classic symptoms, the gallbladder will show inflammation. Therefore, the oral gallbladder X-ray must always be used in combination with the clinical symptoms in determining the presence or absence of gallbladder disease.

A new X-ray test called abdominal ultrasonography has helped doctors diagnose gallstones that were not seen on the oral gallbladder X-ray. This X-ray technique utilizes sound waves to outlines the gallbladder, liver, and bile ducts.

A composite of the sound waves' reflections outlines these organs and body structures. This technique has been especially helpful in establishing a correct diagnosis of a trapped gallstone in the main bile duct. This has enabled patients to receive operative relief sooner and to prevent infectious complications from occurring as a result of that condition.

Surgical Removal of the Gallbladder

When and for what conditions of the gallbladder should it be surgically removed? Individuals who have symptoms indicating gallstones and have X-ray evidence of gallstones should have their gallbladder surgically removed. Formerly the gallstones were removed with the gallbladder being left in. However, many of these patients reformed gallstones and required a second operation for the removal of the gallbladder. Presently the surgical removal of the gallbladder is the operation of choice for gallstones. This operation is known as a cholecystectomy. Individuals who are found to have gallstones by gallbladder X-ray, but who have no symptoms of gallbladder disease, pose a difficult problem for their physician. If the person is less than fifty years of age, elective removal of the gallbladder is recommended. The reason is that one third of these individuals will develop symptoms as a result of their gallstones. If the person is over sixty years of age, the decision regarding surgery is more difficult. Cholecystectomy is more difficult surgery in this age group and is associated with a higher complication rate than in younger individuals.[6]

What about those individuals who have an abnormal gallbladder X-ray but without evidence of gallstones and whose symptoms are suggestive of gallbladder disease? It is important that these individuals are fully evaluated before gallbladder surgery is done. These individuals may have their symptoms because of another digestive disease such as reflux esophagitis, gastritis, or an irritable bowel syndrome.

If the correct diagnosis is not identified before gallbladder surgery is done, some of these people will have disappointing results after their operations.

Unfortunately having your gallbladder surgically removed does not mean that you will not be troubled by gallstone problems again. About 10 percent of individuals will have recurrent gallstones.[7] The gallstones will continue to form within the bile ducts instead of the gallbladder. The recurrent stones can cause the same symptoms as before. If an individual has recurrent gallstones that block the main bile duct, these stones can now be removed without having general surgery. How are these gallstones nonsurgically removed?

Nonsurgical Removal of Gallstones

Using a flexible instrument known as a duodenoscope, a digestive disease specialist can locate the opening of the bile duct as it enters into the beginning of the small intestine, or duodenum. A small catheter is placed through the duodenoscope into this opening and dye is put into the bile duct to confirm the presence of a gallstone. Then a special catheter with a retractable surgical cutting wire is placed in position at the bile duct opening. Electrical current is passed through it and the opening is enlarged. The gallstone can then pass spontaneously or may be removed utilizing a flexible basket. This technique of endoscopic papillotomy has been helpful in many individuals having recurrent gallstones after having their gallbladder surgery.[8]

Is there a new oral therapy for gallstones that works by dissolving them? At the present time there is a gallstone-dissolving agent available.[9] This agent consists of a bile acid known as chenodeoxycholic acid or chenic acid. It works by making the bile more soluble so that the gallstone dissolves. This medication works on gallstones containing mainly cholesterol crystals with little calcium within them. This type of stone is known as a radiolucent stone. Chenic acid is effective, but the main question regarding its usage relates to the need for its continued usage to keep the stones from recurring and the cost effectiveness of this form of treatment. The answers to these questions and others will be determined by continuing medical studies.

Summary

Diseases of the gallbladder are a frequent cause of gastric distress for millions of Americans. Some individuals will have classic gallbladder symptoms, while others will have a diagnosis of gallbladder disease established only after extensive evaluation. The need for gallbladder removal or cholecystectomy remains an important part of the treatment of gallbladder disease. The newer nonsurgical removal of recurrent gallstones has benefited many individuals. The exact place that the gallstone-dissolving agents will have in the treatment of gallstone-related gallbladder disease is continuing to be investigated.

chapter fifteen
Diseases
of the Pancreas

The pancreas is the hidden digestive gland. This organ was the last digestive gland to be discovered by the early scientists. The pancreas serves a dual function. It is an important source of digestive enzymes and it is the source of insulin, which is required to control the body's sugar metabolism. Diseases of the pancreas are being recognized more frequently as a cause of abdominal pain. Cancer of the pancreas is a dreaded disease with a very poor outlook or prognosis. The newer diagnostic instruments and tests have enabled physicians to recognize disorders of the pancreas more easily.

The pancreas is located behind the stomach and the intestines. It is actually located behind the abdominal cavity, in a position that is known as retroperitoneal in medical terms. Because of this location, it has always been difficult to evaluate the pancreas by medical tests. It has only been in the last ten to twelve years that technological advances have allowed physicians to evaluate the pancreas more adequately.[1] For the first time doctors are now able to visualize the pancreas and find abnormalities that were formerly only detected by surgical exploration. This advancement in diagnostic equipment has enabled physicians to treat more effectively individuals with diseases of the pancreas.

The pancreas has a vital role in the digestive process. This gland produces digestive enzymes that are needed for the proper digestion of fats and protein foods. Any disease process that limits this gland's production of these necessary enzymes will result in problems in fat and protein absorption or uptake. Chronic pancreatitis is a disease that is characterized by extensive destruction of the digestive enzyme-producing cells within the pancreas.

Symptoms of Chronic Pancreatitis

Individuals suffering with chronic pancreatitis may show evidence of fat and protein malnutrition.[2] The loss of these two fundamental body requirements will result in weight loss, a decrease in the body's muscle mass and vitamin deficiencies. Many vitamins are fat soluble; that is, they require proper fat absorption for their uptake by the body. Vitamins A, K, D, and E are the fat-soluble vitamins. Therefore, people with chronic pancreatitis and improper fat absorption may demonstrate deficiencies of these vitamins.

Vitamin A is required for proper night vision. Night blindness could result from inadequate absorption of vitamin A. Vitamin K is required for proper blood clotting. A low body level of vitamin K could predispose the body to abnormal bleeding. Bleeding underneath the skin could produce a typical purplish discoloration of the skin. Bleeding from the GI tract, female organs, or the urinary tract can result from a low level of vitamin K. Vitamin D is required for the proper handling of calcium and phosphorus, which are two minerals needed for proper bone strength and structure. Individuals having a low level of vitamin D might have bone pain and softening of the bones. Fractures of the bones might occur from incidents that would not have resulted in broken bones in individuals with a normal level of vitamin D.

Individuals with chronic pancreatitis may complain of severe abdominal pain, diarrhea, and possible evidence of sugar imbalance. The pain associated with chronic pancreatitis is an intense, unremitting pain that is located deep in the abdominal cavity. This pain frequently radiates into the back and is felt between the lower portions of the shoulder blades. The pain of chronic pancreatitis is increased when the patient lies flat on his or her back and is relieved somewhat when the patient bends forward at the hips. Therefore, individuals with severe pain may sleep in a chair in a sitting position. The severity of this pain may require the use of narcotic pain relievers for its relief. Addiction is commonly observed among people with chronic pancreatitis because these medications allow some relief from their terrible painful existence.

Diarrhea is a frequent complaint of people suffering from chronic pancreatitis. This diarrhea results from the improper absorption of fats. The diarrhea is frequently persistent and creates family problems because of its extremely malodorous nature. The bowel movements appear greasy and frothy with a tendency to leave a grease ring around the commode. This type of diarrhea is not controlled with medications normally used for other types of diarrhea. The diarrhea of chronic pancreatitis is controlled with medications that correct the fat malabsorption. These medications contain extracts of the normally produced pancreatic enzymes. These preparations are taken with meals to allow for the proper uptake of fats by the body.

Some individuals with chronic pancreatitis will demonstrate an inability to handle their normal sugar metabolism and have sugar diabetes, or diabetes mellitus. This results from the destruction of the insulin-producing cells within the pancreas by the chronic inflammation. These patients will have the same symptoms as other diabetic patients and may require insulin for the control of their blood sugar.

It is evident that chronic pancreatitis is a severely disabling condition that has a dramatic impact on the life styles of those people suffering from this disease. What are the causes of chronic pancreatitis? Alcohol abuse and gallstone disease are the two most common causes of chronic pancreatitis. Alcohol abuse is the most common cause of chronic pancreatitis in the United States. It is the most frequent cause of chronic pancreatitis in males because of the slightly higher rate of alcoholism in men. A direct toxic effect of the alcohol on the pancreas is the reason why these people develop chronic pancreatitis.[3] The poor diet that many of these chronic drinkers have is another reason why this chronic inflammation of the pancreas results so frequently. Women with chronic pancreatitis may develop it as a result of alcohol abuse, but more frequently it results as a consequence of gallstone disease. The gallstones travel down the main common bile duct and enter the small intestines; this is the common exit for the common bile duct and the pancreatic duct as it enters the small intestine. A gallstone could block the pancreatic duct and cause an acute inflammation of the pancreas, known as acute pancreatitis. Repeated episodes of this sequence could result in chronic inflammation, scarring, and the resultant chronic pancreatitis. (See Illustration 7, page 118.)

Treatment of Chronic Pancreatitis

The treatment of chronic pancreatitis has many facets. Nutritional replacement therapy consists of supplemental pancreatic enzymes to facilitate the absorption of fats and proteins. These enzyme supplements will help correct the diarrhea, weight loss, and muscle wasting that many of these patients exhibit. Vitamin replacements are important to correct or prevent fat soluble vitamin deficiencies. Insulin may be required to control a diabetic state.

The control of the pain associated with chronic pancreatitis is a difficult medical task. If the pain is totally uncontrolled with medications or a narcotic-dependent state results, surgical approaches may be necessary. Surgical removal of parts or all of the pancreas gland have given relief of pain in some patients. If a 95 percent removal of the pancreas is performed, those patients will require all the nutritional supplement measures to maintain their proper fat, protein, and sugar metabolism.

Other individuals suffering from chronic pancreatitis may benefit from a different type of operation. In this operation the pancreatic duct is made to drain directly into a portion of the small intestine, which has been opened and sewn around the pancreatic duct.[4] It is hoped that this operation will allow for better drainage of the pancreatic enzymes into the intestine and improve the absorption of fat and protein. It may also reduce the amount of pain experienced by some of these individuals. The results of this operation vary considerably from patient to patient.

Causes of Acute Pancreatitis

An acute inflammatory condition of the pancreas, known as acute pancreatitis, is a common cause of severe abdominal pain. This digestive disease is being recognized more frequently because of increased awareness of it by physicians. Most cases of acute pancreatitis have a self-limiting illness associated with an eventual recovery, but it may be a life-threatening disease in some individuals.

Alcohol is the most common cause of acute pancreatic inflammation. Most commonly an attack of acute pancreatitis results after a heavy drinking spree. However, the steady consumption of alcohol may result in an attack of acute pancreatitis. Pancreatic inflammation results from a direct effect of the alcohol on the pancreas.

There is a known association relating gallstones to acute pancreatitis. The explanation of how gallstones result in pancreatic inflammation has been previously reviewed in the section dealing with chronic pancreatitis. This cause of acute pancreatitis is more commonly seen in women than men because of their higher incidence of gallstone disease.

Many digestive diseases involving the small intestine may precipitate an attack of acute pancreatitis. A deep peptic ulceration of this part of the small intestine is an unusual cause of acute pancreatic inflammation. Rarely, Crohn's disease of the duodenum could cause acute pancreatitis. Certain diseases that are associated with a high fat content of the blood may cause acute pancreatitis. The increased fat is usually the triglyceride component rather than the cholesterol fraction of the blood. Certain women taking birth control pills will develop this increased triglyceride pattern in their blood. This increase is felt to result as a side effect of the medication. This would predispose the body to a more probable state for the development of acute pancreatitis.

Mumps is an infectious cause of acute pancreatitis. Pancreatitis is rarely associated with mumps in childhood but is frequently seen in association with mumps in adolescence. In most cases of adult onset mumps-related pancreatitis, the pancreatic inflammation is more bothersome than the swelling of the parotid glands. In some patients there is no swelling of the parotid glands and the diagnosis of mumps-related pancreatitis is established by a blood test for the mumps virus.

As previously stated, acute pancreatitis is sometimes a potentially fatal disease. In these cases the pancreatic enzymes excessively disrupt the gland and the blood vessels supplying it. This results in a hemorrhagic or bleeding pancreatic inflammation that is associated with a 50 percent death rate.[5] Fortunately the majority of cases of pancreatitis are not of this variety and respond to therapy.

Treatment of Acute Pancreatitis

The majority of people with acute pancreatitis will benefit from hospitalization. The stomach will be pumped via a gastric tube through the nose so that the pancreas will not be stimulated by the stomach's secretions. This procedure will be continued until the blood tests show that the pancreatic inflammation is subsiding. Most cases resolve in five to seven days. Diet is slowly advanced to include fatty foods. Their absence in the early days after recovery from the acute episode allows for less stimulation of the pancreatic enzyme cells. Depending upon the cause of the acute episode of pancreatitis, appropriate treatment will be given. Elective gallbladder surgery is indicated in individuals with gallstones and repeated attacks of acute pancreatitis. The surgery is performed a couple of months after the acute episode to assure complete resolution of the inflammation within the pancreas. Alcohol usage should be discontinued in those cases where the acute inflammation is believed to result from its use. In those people in whom an abnormal blood fat level is identified, appropriate dietary measures can be taken to reduce it. If an individual is taking birth control pills, they should be discontinued.

Is acute pancreatitis a precursor of chronic pancreatitis? This is a difficult question to answer. It is mainly dependent upon the cause of the acute episode of pancreatitis. People who continue to drink excessive amounts of alcohol and have acute episodes of pancreatitis could develop chronic pancreatitis. Individuals with undiagnosed gallstones as the cause of their repeated attacks of acute pancreatitis will be at an increased risk for the development of a chronic pancreatic inflammation. Most people suffering one attack of acute pancreatic inflammation will not develop chronic pancreatitis on that basis. The habitual injury to the pancreas seems to be the important causative factor in the development of chronic pancreatitis.

Cancer of the Pancreas:
Symptoms and Treatment

Cancer of the pancreas is a malignancy that is difficult to diagnose early and is associated with a terrible prognosis. This cancer is a disease of middle-aged Americans. This disease is rarely seen in individuals younger than forty years of age. Individuals with a family history of pancreatic cancer and patients with chronic pancreatitis and diabetes have an increased risk of developing pancreatic cancer. It is not known how these factors and conditions predispose the body to the development of this malignancy.

The inaccessibility of the pancreas to diagnostic testing and the nonspecific nature of the symptoms of early pancreatic cancer result in the diagnosis being made late in the course of this cancer. This accounts for the poor survival rate among those with this tumor.

What are the symptoms of pancreatic cancer? The majority of people will notice a slow, steady weight loss. This results from their loss of appetite. The persons eat only because they know they should. Some individuals will notice the onset of a vague pain in the middle of their abdomen that may be made worse by lying down. Many of these people have a premonition of impending doom or that something is seriously wrong with them. Depression and abnormal psychological behavior are frequently observed in patients with pancreatic cancer. About half of the individuals will have these mental symptoms.[6] If a middle-aged individual notices any of these symptoms, he or she should consult a doctor immediately. In this way an earlier diagnosis of pancreatic cancer can be made and it is hoped that the survival rate or prognosis will be improved for those suffering from this malignancy.

As the tumor grows, jaundice will usually develop as the bile ducts are blocked by the cancer. More than half of the individuals with pancreatic cancer will have icterus, or yellowish color, of their eyes and skin as a late sign of this disease. Unfortunately, by this time, the tumor is frequently beyond surgical removal.

Summary

In terms of its location, the pancreas is the silent gland of the digestive tract. It has important functions in the maintenance of normal sugar metabolism and fat and protein absorption.

Acute and chronic inflammation of this gland can result in disabling conditions. Cancer of the pancreas has a poor prognosis because of the difficulty of detecting it early. It is hoped that the future will reveal a test that will allow for the early diagnosis of pancreatic cancer. Until that time all middle-aged adults should be aware of the symptoms of early pancreatic cancer. Consult your physician promptly if you notice the presence of any of these symptoms.

chapter sixteen
Viral Hepatitis

Viral hepatitis is an infection of the liver that results in liver cell dysfunction. Most cases of viral hepatitis resolve without complications, but a small percentage of cases may progress to chronic liver disease. There are three viruses that cause hepatitis, and each virus is associated with different possible consequences of this infection. This chapter will review the treatment and preventive aspects of viral hepatitis.

Infectious hepatitis is the viral hepatitis that most commonly causes community-wide epidemics. It is the type of viral hepatitis that most high school and college students and servicemen develop. This type of viral hepatitis is very contagious and mainly spreads as the result of poor personal hygiene practices. The virus is shed in the stools of the infected person, and poor hygienic technique allows for its spread by the hand-to-mouth route. The infected person touches something and the next individual touches the same object and then puts his or her hands into the mouth and becomes exposed to the virus. It is easily seen why this viral infection is so contagious. Serum hepatitis results most commonly after a blood transfusion in which the blood or blood product is contaminated with the causative virus. This type of viral hepatitis was formerly seen only in patients receiving blood transfusions or in hospital personnel who were exposed directly to their blood. The latter may have resulted from a needle puncture of the skin by a nurse, or exposure to the virus by a laboratory technician while drawing blood from a patient with hepatitis. Today serum hepatitis is frequently observed in heroin addicts who share needles. This cause of serum hepatitis has steadily increased over recent years.[1] This type of hepatitis is also being recognized with increased frequency in homosexual males.[2] Recent evidence has shown that this virus can be transmitted through saliva and semen. Intimate contact allows for the passage of the virus by either means of transfer. An individual's sexual contacts are also at risk for developing this type of hepatitis through their intimate contact. The virus that causes this form of hepatitis is not shed in the stools, so the hand-to-mouth mode of transmission is not an important means of transferring this type of hepatitis.

Infectious hepatitis is caused by the virus known as the Type A hepatitis virus. This form of viral hepatitis has an incubation period—the time from the exposure of the virus to the development of symptoms—of fifteen to sixty days. Serum hepatitis is caused by the Type B hepatitis virus and has a longer incubation period than Type A hepatitis. Usually the incubation period is from sixty to 120 days. The difference in the incubation periods was formerly used by physicians to distinguish between the two types of hepatitis.

Today physicians have the availability of blood tests that allow them to distinguish between Type A and Type B hepatitis. It is important to identify the type of hepatitis so that proper preventive and prophylactic measures can be taken. These blood tests also enable blood banks to screen their blood products to determine the presence or absence of Type B hepatitis virus within them. This screening method has resulted in a dramatic decrease in the incidence of posttransfusion hepatitis. Hepatitis can still result after receiving blood products, but the number of cases that result from Type B hepatitis virus has decreased steadily. Presently 10 percent of people that receive a blood transfusion could develop hepatitis as a consequence of it.[3] However, less than 25 percent of those cases will be due to the Type B hepatitis virus.

Symptoms of Acute
Viral Hepatitis

What are the symptoms of acute viral hepatitis? Both Type A and Type B hepatitis have clinical symptoms that are very similar. Before the typical yellowing, or icteric phase, of acute hepatitis occurs, most individuals experience symptoms typical of a viral illness. They complain of weakness, muscular achings, generalized headache, poor appetite, and easy fatigability. Some individuals lose their taste for cigarettes during this time period. A low-grade fever may be seen, but shaking chills are rare. These symptoms last on the average of three to five days before the onset of yellowing of the skin and the whites of the eyes is noticed.

As the yellowing color deepens, the flulike symptoms disappear; the person will look terrible but feel improved. The appetite slowly improves as does energy availability. The majority of individuals will notice a darkening discoloration of their urine during this icteric period. The urine may appear coke-colored. About half of the individuals will notice a generalized itching of the skin during this period of time if their skin is yellow. The yellowish discoloration of the skin may last up to four weeks, but in most patients it clears within a week to ten days. With the disappearance of the skin discoloration, the individual is cured of hepatitis in the majority of cases.

What causes the yellowing of the skin to occur during an episode of acute, hepatitis? The hepatitis virus obstructs the ability of the liver cells to take a pigment, called bilirubin, out of the blood. This pigment collects in the blood and at high levels enters into the skin. The collection of the bilirubin pigment in the skin results in the yellowish coloration. Generalized itching, which many individuals with acute hepatitis have, results from the presence of the pigment within the skin. The kidneys clear this pigment from the blood, and its presence in the urine accounts for its darkened color.

Although most individuals with acute hepatitis experience complete recovery, some people are less fortunate. Occasionally either type of hepatitis virus causes a fulminant or severe hepatitis that may be fatal. In these cases the severe liver injury prohibits the liver from clearing the body's nitrogen waste products as it normally does. Abnormally high blood levels of these substances may adversely affect the functioning of the brain and kidneys. If either organ is severely affected, the outcome may be fatal.

Some cases of viral hepatitis do not resolve completely but display evidence for continued hepatic inflammation.[4] In these individuals the hepatic cell injury continues, and serious damage to the function and structure of the liver can result. This continued liver inflammation is called chronic active hepatitis. This complication occurs more frequently with Type B hepatitis than with Type A hepatitis. It is a rare case of Type A hepatitis that does not resolve completely. It is important to recognize this possible complication of viral hepatitis because this condition may result in cirrhosis of the liver. The identification of chronic active hepatitis as an important consequence of viral hepatitis has only been achieved in the last decade and a half. Presently it is impossible to predict which cases of acute hepatitis will progress to chronic active liver disease. The main concern has been to find a way to prevent those unfortunate individuals who have chronic active hepatitis from progressing to cirrhosis of the liver. At the present time studies are underway to evaluate various treatment methods for chronic active hepatitis. It is hoped that these studies will demonstrate a means to prevent progression of this liver disease to cirrhosis.

Treatment
for Acute Viral Hepatitis

Should there be any dietary or physical activity restrictions for patients having acute viral hepatitis? It is important that individuals consume a balanced diet with no food restrictions unless outlined by their physician. A diet high in calories and protein is necessary to allow the liver cells to regenerate and clear the inflammation from within them. In some cases of severe hepatitis the protein content of the diet will be limited to help prevent any increase of the harmful nitrogen products in the blood. In those cases the liver injury prohibits the normal clearing of those substances from the blood and may result in abnormal functioning of the brain or kidneys. Remember, unless specifically instructed by your physician, consume a balanced diet of high caloric and protein content.

There is some debate in medical circles concerning which is the proper activity for patients having acute viral hepatitis. Some physicians recommend strict bedrest for their patients until there is clearing of the yellowish discoloration of the skin. Other doctors allow their patients to ambulate at will but advise them to avoid strenuous or fatiguing circumstances. The prevailing view of most physicians is to allow full ambulation, but they follow the individuals' progress closely. If there is worsening of the liver functions, bedrest would then be recommended.

Preventing the Spread
of Viral Hepatitis

What precautions should the family members take to prevent the development of viral hepatitis? When should family members receive a shot to help in the prevention of acute hepatitis? It is important to know the type of virus that is responsible for causing the episode of acute hepatitis. The recommendations will vary according to the responsible viral agent. Good personal hygiene is important for both types of hepatitis virus, but it is especially important with Type A hepatitis because of the highly contagious nature of that virus in regard to the hand-to-mouth method of spread. It is important during epidemics to stress at school proper personal hygiene technique, including vigorous hand washings. The same measures are important to prevent the spread of Type A hepatitis through a family household.

People living in the same house with a patient with Type A hepatitis are exposed to the virus by the time that individual becomes yellow. Family members may be infected and already in the incubation period of the hepatitis infection. Those household contacts should receive a Gamma globulin shot. Gamma globulin is a commercially made preparation that contains human antibodies against the viral agent. This preparation is given in the form of a shot in the buttocks. It is hoped that this antibody preparation will prevent an episode of acute Type A hepatitis from occurring, and that if an attack of hepatitis occurs, it will be a milder form. There may be evidence of liver function abnormalities, but the individual may not become yellow if hepatitis occurs after the Gamma globulin prophylaxis.

With schoolwide epidemics of Type A hepatitis, the Gamma globulin shot should be administered only to the neighborhood friends of those with hepatitis. Schoolwide inoculation programs are less effective than the neighborhood prophylactic approach. This is because of the more immediate and intimate contact with close friends.

At the present time there is no immunization shot or vaccine that can be given on a national scale to prevent the development of Type A hepatitis. It is hoped that the future will show the development of such a vaccine.

What should be done to prevent the transmission of Type B hepatitis to other individuals? As previously discussed, the transmission of Type B hepatitis appears to be mainly by exposure to the blood, saliva, or semen of the individual with hepatitis. Therefore, hospital personnel must be very careful to prevent such accidental exposure to the blood of those individuals with Type B hepatitis. Heroin users must be aware of the dangers of sharing needles with a person known to have Type B hepatitis. Loved ones of individuals with Type B hepatitis may contact the virus by intimate contact or sexual relations.

Both the regular Gamma globulin and a special type of Gamma globulin that contains a very high level of antibodies against Type B hepatitis virus are effective in reducing the transmission of Type B hepatitis. As would be expected, the high titer Gamma globulin preparation offers more protection. Several national studies have demonstrated that the special type of Gamma globulin is effective in preventing the transmission of Type B hepatitis in spouses and hospital personnel.[5] Unfortunately this protection lasts for only six months and then the person could develop hepatitis. A shot is recommended for household members and other intimate contacts of those individuals with known Type B hepatitis.

Recently, a new hepatitis B vaccine was released for use in the United States. Studies have shown this vaccine to be safe and effective in preventing Type B acute hepatitis.[6] The main application of this virus has been to vaccinate health care personnel, homosexual males, and household or sexual contacts of individuals known to have Type B hepatitis infection.

A third type of hepatitis virus has been recognized. As you would expect, it has been named the Type C, or non-A, non-B, hepatitis virus. This viral agent has been shown to be responsible for the majority of cases of hepatitis that result from receiving blood or blood products. An important feature that helps to distinguish this type of hepatitis is its much shorter incubation period. Some cases of Type C hepatitis have resulted only two weeks after the exposure to the virus. This type of hepatitis virus is associated with the development of chronic liver disease, as is Type B hepatitis. Much more information is still being gained about this new hepatitis virus and the consequences of its infection.

Cirrhosis or end-stage liver disease can result from an episode of acute viral hepatitis. In some of these cases that progress to cirrhosis, the individuals did not know that they had hepatitis because they did not have yellowing of the skin. The virus causes a subclinical hepatitis that persisted and resulted in cirrhosis. Chapter 17 will discuss in detail cirrhosis of the liver.

Summary

Viral hepatitis remains a common liver ailment. Most cases will resolve without complications, but some individuals develop chronic or end-stage liver disease from a viral hepatitis infection. It is hoped that the future will show the presence of a vaccine for both types of viral hepatitis. Until that time the preventive measures outlined in this chapter can help reduce the number of cases of viral hepatitis.

chapter seventeen

Cirrhosis
of the Liver

Cirrhosis of the liver, or a scarred, abnormally functioning liver, is one of the leading causes of death in middle-aged Americans. This liver disease can result from many different causes, but it most commonly results from chronic alcoholic consumption. This disease is associated with a high death rate and a high rate of personal disability.

Cirrhosis of the liver could result from either a single severe episode of liver injury or from a chronic damaging insult to the liver. Viral hepatitis is an example of a single episode of a liver injury that could result in the development of liver cirrhosis. Alcohol is the most common example of a substance causing continuous liver injury that could progress to cirrhosis.

In a cirrhotic liver the normal architecture is replaced by fibrous scarring and disorganization of the liver cells. This altered liver structure results in abnormal liver function. This abnormal liver function is responsible for the symptoms, the physical findings, and the complications that people with cirrhosis have.

Symptoms of Cirrhosis

One of the most common symptoms experienced by individuals with cirrhosis is the deterioration from a state of good health. These individuals do not feel like eating, feel weak and tired, and are unable to perform tasks that were formerly routine. These individuals lose muscle mass from their shoulders and hip girdles as a consequence of malnutrition. A large protuberant abdomen or pot-belly could result from the collection of fluid within the abdominal cavity. This fluid within the abdominal cavity is known as ascites, or ascitic fluid. Association of this ascitic fluid with cirrhosis of the liver has been recognized since Hippocrates, the first physician. The collection of fluid within the abdominal cavity was formerly known as dropsy in the early 1900s. Ascitic fluid results as a consequence of the abnormal liver functioning. This fluid gives the individual a false sense of security because his or her weight increases due to its presence. The weight may increase, but the muscle mass decreases. This muscle wasting, coupled with the large protuberant abdomen, gives some individuals a very characteristic appearance.

People with cirrhosis of the liver may notice the onset of a hand tremor. The tremor may become so severe as to cause problems with eating or daily personal hygiene. The tremor results from abnormal protein substances, present in the blood, which affect the normal functioning of the brain. These protein substances, which are normally cleared from the blood by a healthy liver, cannot be removed by the cirrhotic liver. The resultant abnormal brain function is called an encephalopathy. This liver-related encephalopathy can cause mental confusion, restless nights, and improper thinking. People will notice they have difficulty doing addition or subtraction, become confused about the exact date or place where they are, and have daytime or nighttime frightening dreams. Unfortunately this encephalopathy can progress to coma and death. This liver-related brain disorder is a major cause of personal disability and death in individuals with cirrhosis.[1] Ways to prevent and treat this liver-related encephalopathy will be discussed later in this chapter.

Many people with cirrhosis will be found to be anemic. This anemia can result from a variety of causes. Poor dietary intake may allow for the presence of a folate or folic acid deficiency. This situation can result in an anemic amount of red blood cells being produced by the body. Liver disease may allow for an abnormal metabolism of vitamin B-12 and iron, which can contribute to the anemic state. The anemia will contribute to the individual's weakness and easy fatigability.

Individuals with cirrhosis can have skin changes that are secondary to their chronic liver disease. Some people will notice the yellowing of their skin. This jaundice does not occur as frequently as with an acute hepatitis. Indeed, severe jaundice in a cirrhotic patient would usually indicate a worsening of the liver function. Some individuals will notice liver spots, which are small, flat, reddish-discolored skin areas. Some individuals with liver spots will notice a redness of the palms of their hands. Both the liver spots and the palmer erythema, or redness, are caused by the liver's inability to normally metabolize sex hormones. Some cirrhotic patients will notice the presence of narrow white bands across their fingernail beds. These white lines result from a low blood albumin level. Serum albumin is the main blood protein made by the liver, and a chronically injured liver is not capable of making the normal amount of albumin. The nail bed changes reflect the abnormal rate at which albumin is made.

Many endocrine or hormonal changes can occur as a result of the diseased liver's inability to properly metabolize the hormones that are present in the bloodstream. Frequently, male cirrhotics will notice tenderness of their breasts. This painful swelling results from an increase in the amount of breast tissue present. This change, called gynecomastia, occurs as a consequence of the abnormal hormone metabolism. Many male individuals with cirrhosis will complain of a decreased sexual drive and impotency. These unfortunate changes result from the abnormal endocrine state. There is little that can be done to increase the sex drive or correct the presence of impotency in these individuals.

It is easily seen that individuals with cirrhosis have multiple symptoms and physical findings that result in physical disability and necessitate changes in their life styles.

Complications Resulting from Cirrhosis

There are many complications associated with cirrhosis of the liver. Some of these complications are life threatening and may result in the ultimate demise of the individual. One of the most dramatic complications of liver cirrhosis is massive bleeding from the upper GI tract. This bleeding can result from the rupture of large veins that are present in the lining of the esophagus. These large veins are called varices. Normal individuals or individuals without cirrhosis do not have these large veins present in their esophagus. These large veins result from the altered blood flow through the cirrhotic liver. This type of bleeding is associated with a high death rate.

If an individual survives an episode of variceal bleeding, he or she may be a candidate for an operation that it is hoped will prevent any further episodes of such bleeding. The reason this operation is performed is to decrease the risk of another severe episode of variceal bleeding. Cirrhotics who have had one variceal bleeding episode are at increased risk to have another severe bleeding episode that they may not survive. The operation performed for the prevention of future variceal bleeding is called a portal-caval shunt. During this operation, the main venous blood supply to the liver is redirected away from the liver. The purpose of this operation is to decrease the pressure within the esophageal varices and render them less susceptible to bleeding. Unfortunately, some of the individuals having this shunt operation will develop encephalopathy after surgery. Recently modifications of the original shunt operation have increased the efficiency and the prevention of future variceal bleeding episodes and have been associated with a lower incidence of postoperative encephalopathy.

It is important that individuals with cirrhosis experiencing an episode of upper GI bleeding have the diagnosis of esophageal variceal bleeding properly excluded. An upper GI X-ray will only demonstrate the presence or absence of esophageal varices and will not determine whether or not they are actively bleeding. An upper GI endoscopy examination is much more helpful in determining the exact cause of the bleeding. This examination allows for the visual inspection of the lining of the esophagus. If there is evidence of variceal bleeding, the individual might be a candidate for a shunt operation after recovering from the acute bleeding episode.

If the shunt operations are usually successful in preventing future episodes of variceal bleeding, why are they not done to prevent bleeding initially? This seems like a very logical question. However, studies have shown that shunts done on individuals who have not had an episode of variceal bleeding live shorter lives than those who do not have the shunt performed.[2] Therefore, the shunt operations are done only to prevent further episodes of bleeding from the esophagus and are not done on individuals not having a previously documented episode of variceal hemorrhage.

Hepatic encephalopathy and coma are complications of cirrhosis that may result in the death of an individual. As previously stated, these complications result from the diseased liver being unable to handle properly certain protein substances that are present within the bloodstream. Prevention of this complication is directed at reducing the dietary protein intake and decreasing the body's ability to make potentially dangerous protein or nitrogen substances. People are given a low-protein diet with strict dietary instructions on how to calculate the exact amount of protein taken in daily. A low-protein diet is not very tasty or palatable, but these individuals adhere to it because of the noted improvement in their symptoms.

The bacteria within the large bowel produces nitrogen products that may increase the level of the encephalopathy. Therefore, physicians can use medications that will reduce the number of these bacteria in an attempt to improve the encephalopathy. Neomycin is a nonabsorbed antibiotic that has been used to reduce the number of colonic bacteria and lower the blood level of these potentially harmful nitrogen products. This antibiotic was the first successful medication to be used in the treatment of hepatic encephalopathy. Unfortunately the long-term usage of this drug has been associated with potential hearing loss and possible kidney damage. Neomycin has now been replaced by a nonabsorbable sugar that is equally effective in the therapy of the liver encephalopathy. Lactulose is the name of the sugar that is presently being used. The sugar works by rendering the bowel less capable of absorbing or taking up the harmful nitrogen products of the large bowel bacteria. There have been no reported serious side effects of this new treatment modality. The sugar does produce some diarrhea, but this can be controlled by adjusting the dosage.

An important liver-kidney relationship may exist in some people with cirrhosis. In some individuals the kidneys stop functioning properly. In this condition the kidneys appear normal and demonstrate no abnormal changes of their structure. The exact reason why these normal-appearing kidneys stop functioning in some individuals with cirrhosis is not fully understood. Commonly this type of liver-kidney failure is not responsive to treatment and results in the death of those individuals.[3] This is one of the most dreaded complications of liver cirrhosis. This complication is known as the hepatorenal syndrome.

The collection of ascitic fluid in the abdominal cavity is also a complication of cirrhosis. This fluid is so frequently

observed in cirrhotic patients, its presence implies a less severe liver disease. The ascitic fluid is commonly associated
with evidence of other extra fluid collecting within the body.
This extra fluid may result in edema, swelling of the ankles
or feet, or fluid collecting within the chest cavity or lungs.
The treatment of this extra body fluid is directed at reducing
the amount of fluids taken in daily and giving medications
that may help eliminate this fluid.

Treatment for Cirrhosis

Fluid restriction is the main treatment of ascitic fluid. People
with cirrhosis must be instructed on the careful management
of their daily fluid intake. Many cirrhotic patients may have
to have their daily fluid intake limited to less than one or
one-and-a-half quarts of fluid. Salt or sodium restriction is
also important in reducing the fluid that individuals take in
their daily diet. The combination of the low sodium or salt
content of the diet, coupled with the protein restriction,
makes eating a task rather than a joy for many individuals
with cirrhosis. However, the effectiveness of the dietary regimen makes it easier to accept.

    A variety of medications that can be given to control
the ascitic fluid are available. These various medications
work by different means to remove the excess fluid and
water from the body. These medications should be used con-
currently with fluid and salt restriction for the best response.
The majority of patients will notice an improvement of their
ascitic fluid with this treatment. The removal or lessening of
the ascites and edema will allow for increased mobility by
these individuals.

    Rarely, a patient with cirrhosis and ascites is
unresponsive to all forms of therapy. What can be done for
these individuals? A new operation that can be performed
under local anesthesia holds new hope for these individuals.
With this procedure a tube is inserted into the abdominal
cavity and run up underneath the skin to the neck area. The

other end of the tube is then placed into a large vein in the neck. This conduit system allows for the ascitic fluid to drain from the abdominal cavity into the body's circulatory system. The syphon effect is responsible for the movement of the fluid. Once the ascitic fluid is in the bloodstream, it is cleared by the kidneys and excreted. This new technique is being evaluated to determine its effectiveness and safety.

All the described complications occur most commonly in cirrhotic patients who are in the end-stages of their liver disease. Many people with cirrhosis of the liver will have stable liver functions and not experience any problems for prolonged time periods. It is impossible for any physician to predict which person with cirrhosis will, or when they will, have a decompensation of their liver function and become more likely to develop one of the complications of cirrhosis.

Because of the chronic scarring and inflammation within the liver, there is a small chance that a percentage of individuals with cirrhosis will develop a primary tumor or cancer of the liver. This complication is more likely to occur in a liver having cirrhosis secondary to a viral infection than in one with cirrhosis secondary to alcohol abuse.[4] One clue to its presence would be the sudden deterioration in a cirrhotic's condition that was formerly stable and responding to therapy. It is important to state that most cirrhotics will not be shown to have a primary liver tumor as the cause of this change in their health.

It is recommended that all cirrhotic patients take a vitamin preparation to ensure getting their necessary vitamin requirements. With the dietary restrictions imposed on some individuals with cirrhosis it is easily seen why their diet would not possibly contain the necessary daily vitamins. A pharmacist would be able to assist you in selecting the correct vitamin supplement.

Finally, experimental work is being done on a liver machine, similar to the kidney dialysis machine, which would take the place of the diseased liver and remove various noxious substances from the blood. This work is only in the preliminary stages and has been fraught with disappointments.

It is hoped that the future will bring a liver machine that will be able to prolong the lives of millions of individuals with cirrhosis of the liver.

We hope the incidence of cirrhosis will decrease in the future. A vaccine that will eliminate viral hepatitis would certainly reduce some of the cases.[5] If the consumption of alcohol were decreased, the incidence of cirrhosis would most certainly be lower. Unfortunately the number of people abusing alcohol seems to be increasing. This is especially true in high school students. It is possible that cirrhosis will be recognized in individuals at an earlier age if this trend does not reverse itself.

Summary

Cirrhosis is an unfortunate and severely disabling liver disease that has many causes and many dreaded complications. Social reform in regard to the usage of alcohol is one way in which the number of people suffering from this end-stage liver disease could be reduced. Time will show us the trend and results.

chapter eighteen

Cancer of the GI Tract

Cancers of the digestive tract result in more deaths than cancers of any other organ system. The majority of cancers of the digestive system respond poorly to therapy and have a poor prognosis. Fortunately, the number of cases reported by cancer registries has decreased recently.[1]

Cancer of the colon, or the large intestine and rectum, is the most common malignancy of the digestive tract. Cancer of the gland ranks in the top four types of cancers that individuals develop. The risk of developing a cancer of the colon steadily increases with age, and most cancers of the colon are diagnosed in people over the age of 60.[2]

Causes of Cancer
of the Colon

Cancer of the colon may occur sporadically or be found with unfortunate predictability in certain families.[3] The family genes may predispose individuals to the development of colon cancer in some way. This does not mean that if a brother or sister is found to have cancer of the colon, you will be at an increased risk of developing a colon cancer. The increased risk would exist only in those families where the mother or father, some of the aunts and uncles, and other brothers and sisters are known to have a cancer of the colon. Women with a history of cancer of the uterus and a family member having a history of cancer of the colon are probably at greater risk of developing a cancer of the colon than other members of the family.

Cancer of the colon occurs more frequently in highly industrialized countries than in underdeveloped societies. Why this difference exists between such countries is not known with certainty. Speculations to explain this difference have included a possible exposure to pollutants that may cause cancer, differences in the composition of the diet, and the differences of the type of bacteria found within the large intestine.[4] The role of the diet in the prevention of colon cancer revolves around the data showing that people living in countries where a high-fiber diet is regularly consumed have a lower incidence of colon cancer than individuals consuming a low-fiber diet regularly. The high-fiber diet causes a faster movement of the food through the digestive system, allowing for the bowel lining to be exposed to potential cancer-causing agents for less time. This is believed to explain the decreased incidence of colon cancer in people regularly consuming a high-fiber diet. This observation is the reason why millions of Americans have changed their diets to include high-fiber foods. All digestive disease experts are hopeful that this dietary regimen will actually decrease the number of new colon cancers they will be seeing in the future.

There is some information suggesting that the beef content of the diet is somehow related to the increased incidence of colon cancer. This information suggests that the beef undergoes transformation while within the digestive system and becomes a potential cancer-causing agent in certain individuals. Pure vegetarians should therefore have a lower incidence of cancer of the large intestine. Further studies are needed to completely substantiate this finding.

Symptoms of Cancer of the Colon

What symptoms would a patient with a cancer of the large intestine have? The majority of individuals with cancer of the colon will notice the presence of blood in their bowel movements, weight loss, signs of anemia, and a change in their bowel habits. Bleeding from a cancer of the large bowel may be falsely thought to be due to bleeding from hemorrhoids. Blood in the stools occurring in adults should be considered due to cancer until proven otherwise. At the first sign of rectal bleeding the individual should consult a physician so that proper tests can be done to exclude the presence of a tumor. Undue delay in this regard should be avoided.

Frequently a patient with cancer of the colon notices a change in his or her bowel habits. Constipation may occur as a result of a tumor blocking the passage of material through the large intestine. Constipation developing in a middle-aged individual who formerly had regular bowel movements requires medical evaluation. This is especially true if blood is noticed within the stools.

About one third of people with cancer of the colon will be found to be iron deficient and have an anemia.[5] This iron deficiency anemia results from the bleeding of the cancer within the large intestine. This anemia may result in weakness, fatigability, and shortness of breath.

Diagnosis and Treatment
of Cancer of the Colon

Most individuals with cancer of the colon will have surgery in an attempt to be cured of their malignancy. The effectiveness of this operation will depend upon the size of the tumor and how long the tumor was present before the diagnosis was made. The longer a cancer is present within the colon, the greater chance there is that the tumor will have spread to other parts of the body or that metastases will have occurred. Colon cancers are typically spread to the lymph nodes adjacent to the large intestine and to the liver. A larger cancer of the colon will have a greater chance of developing metastases than a smaller cancer of the large bowel.

Some individuals will be cured of their cancer with surgical removal. Other less fortunate people will have the operation done only to prevent complete bowel blockage by the tumor. Today there are many different drugs that are being used to retard the growth of cancers after an operation has been performed. The use of drugs to control cancers is known as chemotherapy. Chemotherapy offers hope to many of these individuals. Unfortunately only half of the people with a cancer of the large bowel will live for more than five years. This represents an improvement over the dismal 20 percent that was formerly seen.[6]

The hope is that there will be more and more earlier cancers of the colon found by the use of the annual proctoscopic examination and the yearly physical exam, and that the early cancers of the large bowel will be responsive to therapy and be associated with a better survival rate. All adults over the age of forty, or all individuals with a family history of colon cancer, should have an annual physical exam and proctoscopic evaluation. The future may show some new promise in regard to the role that dietary measures have in the prevention of colon cancer. Long-term studies are presently underway to determine the exact relationship of dietary fiber in the prevention and cause of colon cancer.

Stomach cancer is the second most frequent malignancy of the GI tract.[7] In recent years the recognition of new cases of cancer of the stomach has been decreasing in the United States.[8] The reason for the decreasing incidence of stomach cancer in the United States is not known. All digestive specialists are hopeful that the trend will continue, however. Cancer of the stomach is associated with a dismal cure rate. Most people with stomach cancer seek medical advice only after symptoms have persisted for some time. Unfortunately many of these people are found to have advanced stomach cancer when medically evaluated.[9] If improvement is to be made in the cure and survival of stomach cancer patients, more early tumors of the stomach must be found.

In Japan mass screening examinations are done routinely on everyone because of the high rate of stomach cancer observed in that country. This examination includes an endoscopic examination of the lining of the stomach. Because of this screening procedure, one third of all cancers of the stomach are found to be early malignancies.[10] Early cancer of the stomach has a much better cure rate and survival rate than late or advanced gastric cancer. Since this technique of mass screening is not available in America, other methods must be used to detect the presence of an early cancer of the stomach. The most likely method is education of the people in regard to the importance of their symptoms of gastric dysfunction. Any persistent stomach pain, a sensation of being full sooner with eating the same amount of food, a loss of the taste for meats, and stomach discomfort after eating may be signs of cancer of the stomach. These symptoms, if persistent, should be brought to the attention of your physician immediately.

Certain individuals will be at an increased risk of developing cancer of the stomach. People who have the normal healthy stomach lining replaced by a thin or atrophic lining of the stomach will be at an increased risk of developing cancer. This condition is known as chronic atrophic gastritis. Up to 10 percent of individuals with atrophic gastritis can develop a cancer of the stomach.[11] The majority of the cases of atrophic gastritis are due to unknown causes, but all people with pernicious anemia will have an atrophic gastritis. Therefore, certain people with pernicious anemia will be found to have a gastric cancer. The stomach tumors are usually detected ten or more years after the diagnosis of pernicious anemia is made. These individuals should be closely followed and considered for endoscopic examinations of their stomach. In this way early signs of gastric cancer may be detected. It is hoped that this follow-up will detect the early cancers and afford a better prognosis to these individuals. All individuals with pernicious anemia who have not seen their physicians for some time should contact them so that proper evaluation of their stomach can be accomplished.

Cancer of the stomach that is found late in its course will be surgically cured in only a small percentage of the cases. In over half of the patients with advanced gastric cancer, an inoperable tumor will be found at the time of surgery.[12] Unfortunately chemotherapy offers little hope to those people with advanced cancer of the stomach.

The main hope for improved survival with gastric cancer remains an improvement in the detection rate of early cancer of the stomach. Individuals must be aware that unexplained gastric distress may be a symptom of early gastric cancer. I would recommend that all individuals over the age of forty with unexplained persistent gastric symptoms consult their physicians.

Cancer of the pancreas has been reviewed in Chapter 15. This gastrointestinal malignancy has a poor prognosis and high mortality rate. The main problem with cancers of the pancreas has been the nonspecific nature of the early symptoms and the inaccessibility of the gland to diagnostic studies. Newer diagnostic tests have enabled physicians to diagnose pancreatic cancer but not before the majority of these cancers are widespread. It is hoped that the future will bring a new diagnostic test that will detect early pancreatic cancer.

Cancer of the gastrointestinal tract remains a major source of morbidity for thousands of Americans. A reduction of the number of advanced cancers could possibly be achieved with more regular checkups and prompt consultation with a physician regarding unexplained and persistent GI symptoms. Americans must become more aware of the importance and significance of unremitting GI distress.

chapter nineteen

Newer Diagnostic and Treatment Methods in Digestive Disease

Great advancement in the diagnostic capabilities of the digestive disease specialist has been made with the use of the newer flexible fiberoptic instruments. These instruments utilize a light source that is transmitted through flexible light fibers. These fibers are placed in sophisticated instruments that enable the physician to examine the lining of virtually every digestive tract organ. These instruments permit the doctor to obtain tissue samples that can then be examined under the microscope for a pathological diagnosis. Photographs obtained with either a 35 millimeter, Polaroid, or movie camera can be used to document the findings at the time of the examination. These flexible diagnostic instruments are called endoscopes. Those instruments used for the examination of the lining of the colon are called colonoscopes. The instruments used for the inspection of the stomach and duodenum are known as gastroduodenoscopes. Endoscopes utilized for the inspection of the gullet, or esophagus, are knows as esophagoscopes. The procedure by which the colon is examined is called a colonoscopy. Upper GI endoscopy is the procedure by which the esophagus, stomach, and duodenum are examined endoscopically.

In Chapter 2 upper GI endoscopy was discussed in detail. How the patient was prepared for this procedure, how the physician readied the patient for this diagnostic test, and the process by which the doctor performed the inspection of the upper gastrointestinal tract was reviewed. Colonoscopy, or the endoscopic examination of the large intestine, requires a different preparation, and this procedure has both diagnostic and treatment capabilities. When might an individual require colonoscopy, how is the individual prepared, and how is this procedure usually done?

When and How a Colonoscopy Is Performed

The visual inspection of the colon with an endoscope may be performed for many different reasons. It may be required to confirm an abnormal finding on a barium enema, or done because the barium enema did not give an answer for a clinical problem. If the X-ray study demonstrated a suspected tumor or cancer of the colon, showed a single or multiple polyps of the large bowel, a narrowed area or stricture, or a fistula tract connecting the colon to an organ, colonoscopy would yield valuable information to confirm these findings. In addition to the visual confirmation of these pathological conditions, tissue sampling would give a pathological diagnosis of the existing medical problem. This information would be helpful in the planning of the treatment of these conditions.

If an individual has a normal barium enema examination of the colon but had lower GI bleeding or a history of colon cancer or a history of long-standing inflammatory bowel disease or an unexplained iron deficiency anemia, colonoscopy may be done to assist in establishing a diagnosis. Colonoscopy with biopsy, or the taking of large bowel tissue samples, has been helpful in following an individual after a cancer has been surgically removed. In this way a local recurrence of the tumor may be detected. By the same technique an early cancer of the colon may be detected in an individual with long-standing ulcerative colitis. In regard to people with an unexplained lower GI bleed or iron deficiency anemia, certain abnormalities of the blood vessels of the colon may be detected by colonoscopy and not barium enema.

It is evident that colonoscopy has a varied but important role in the diagnosis of digestive disease. This endoscopic procedure has important treatment capabilities, too. Colonoscopic polypectomy, or the removal of a colonic polyp with the colonoscope, has saved many individuals from the need for surgery. Formerly colon polyps were able to be removed only by abdominal surgery. All polyps of the colon cannot be removed by the colonoscopic technique, however. There are two types of colon polyps. The first type is a flat growth off the lining of the bowel, known as a sessile polyp. This type of polyp can usually not be removed with the colonoscope because of its contact with the bowel wall. The second type of polyp has a stalk from which the polyp protrudes off the lining of the large intestine. This type is known as a pedunculated colon polyp. This type of polyp may be removed with the colonoscope.

Removing Colon Polyps

Why is there a need to remove colon polyps? How is it done with the colonoscope? Polyps of the colon vary in their makeup. Certain types of colon polyps have been known to be premalignant in characteristic.[1] That is, cancer may develop in certain types of colon polyps over the years. This relationship is referred to as the colon polyp-cancer sequence.[2] Therefore, if a polyp of the colon is detected, a tissue sample

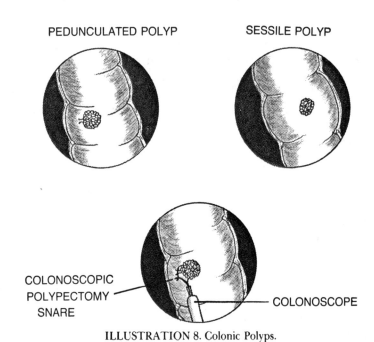

PEDUNCULATED POLYP   SESSILE POLYP

COLONOSCOPIC
POLYPECTOMY
SNARE   COLONOSCOPE

ILLUSTRATION 8. Colonic Polyps.

or biopsy will determine the type of polyp it is. If the polyp
can be removed with the colonoscope, a future cancer may
have been eliminated.[3] Individuals with a history of multiple
colon polyps can now be evaluated periodically with the
colonoscope to determine the presence of new polyps, to remove those polyps that require it, and to obtain tissue
samples of the nonremovable polyps in order to determine
early cancer changes. In this way, certain individuals, at a
higher risk for the development of colon cancer, may be prevented from developing advanced colon cancer.

   If a colon polyp is found that can be removed with
the colonoscope, how is it done? A wire snare, with a loop on
one end, is passed through the colonoscope and adjusted
around the colonic polyp. Electrical current is placed
through this snare and the polyp is severed. This current has
the ability to coagulate, or stop the bleeding, at the

polypectomy site. The polyp is retrieved for review under the microscope to determine its tissue makeup. There is no pain sensation with this technique.

Before a colonoscopy can be performed, the colon must be prepared for the procedure. This will require the removal of the existing digestive residue by laxatives and enemas. In addition, the diet must be limited to clear liquids for a day or two before the procedure to prevent further residue from accumulating within the large intestine. Various combinations of laxatives and enemas have been used to cleanse the colon. The exact preparation for colonoscopy will vary, dependent upon the physician's preference. Generally a typical colonoscopy prep will require twenty-four to forty-eight hours before the procedure can be performed.

Recently a new type of colonic preparation has been utilized by some physicians performing colonoscopy. This preparation requires the drinking of one to two quarts of salt solution within a short time period. This solution allows for a rapid cleansing of the colon. However, individuals vary in their ability to drink this solution in such a short time period. Also the salt content of the preparation may be of concern in the case of certain individuals with severe heart disease. Finally, the efficiency of this new preparation has to be determined by comparative studies.

How a Colonoscopy Is Performed

Once the patient is prepared for colonoscopy, how is the procedure done? The individual is usually given some form of sedative. This medication may be given in a shot intramuscularly or directly into a vein before the colonoscopy. The medication is given to relax or sedate the individual so his or her perception of abdominal discomfort is reduced. As the colonoscope advances from the anus through the large intestine, air is inflated within the colon to ease its passsage. The air can cause abdominal discomfort and cramps. As the colonoscope advances around the curves or flexures of the colon, similar discomfort may be perceived. (See Illustration 1, page 3) The sedative medication will help the tolerance of both causes of abdominal discomfort. As the instrument is withdrawn from the large bowel, the patient usually notices relief of this discomfort.

A shorter version of the colonoscope is now available to be used in the performance of the sigmoidoscopy examination. This new instrument is known as a flexible sigmoidoscope. Flexible sigmoidoscopy affords some important advantages over the conventional rigid sigmoidoscope. First the amount of colon that can be examined is greater with the flexible instrument and, therefore, the yield of information is larger. Secondly the majority of individuals who have had both types of sigmoidoscopic examinations prefer the flexible evaluation. Patient tolerance and cooperation is important with sigmoidoscopy. The preparation of the individual is the same for both types of sigmoidoscopic examinations. One or two enemas immediately before the examination will enable the sigmoid colon to be evaluated in most individuals. Sigmoidoscopy has been reviewed in Chapter 10. As stated before, the most important thing for the individual to do is to relax during sigmoidoscopy. As the individual relaxes, so does their colon, and the sigmoidoscopic examination is performed more easily and more quickly.

In Chapter 14 a newer nonsurgical removal of gallstones has been discussed. The instrument used during this procedure is known as a duodenoscope. This same instrument has provided valuable information in the diagnosis of pancreatic disease. Utilizing a duodenoscope, the physician places a small cannula through the instrument into the opening of the bile ducts. Dye is then injected into the pancreatic duct and X-rays are taken. This diagnostic study is known as E.R.C.P., or endoscopic retrograde cholangio-pancreatography. E.R.C.P. has greatly enhanced the diagnostic capabilities of physicians regarding pancreatic disease and their therapy.

Summary

Technological advances that have occurred within the last decade and a half have enabled improvement in the diagnosis of gastrointestinal disease. The flexible endoscopes have enabled physicians to examine virtually every digestive tract organ. They have greatly enhanced the diagnostic and treatment capabilities of digestive disease specialists.

chapter twenty
References

Chapter 1

1. Morton I. Grossman, "Control of Gastric Secretion," in *Gastrointestinal Disease*, 2nd. ed., eds. Marvin H Sleisenger and John S. Fordtran (Philadelphia: W. B. Saunders Company, 1978), pp. 640–659.
2. Ibid.
3. Ibid.
4. A. Bogoch, ed., *Gastroenterology* (New York: McGraw-Hill, 1973).
5. Grossman, "Control of Gastric Secretion."
6. Graham H. Jeffries, "Gastritis," in *Gastrointestinal Dis ease*, 2nd. ed., eds. Marvin H. Sleisenger and John S

Fordtran (Philadelphia: W. B. Saunders Company, 1978), pp. 733–743.

7. Ibid.

8. H. W. Davenport, "Salicylate damage to the gastric mucosal barrier," *New Eng. J. Med.* 276 (1970), 1307.

Chapter 2

1. Jon Isenberg, Charles T. Richardson, and John S. Fordtran, "Pathogenesis of Peptic Ulcer," in *Gastrointestinal Disease*, 2nd ed., eds. Marvin H. Sleisenger and John S. Fordtran (Philadelphia: W. B. Saunders Company, 1978), pp. 792–806.

2. Richard A. L. Sturdevant and John H. Walsh, "Duodenal Ulcer," in *Gastrointestinal Disease*, 2nd ed., eds. Marvin H. Sleisenger and John S. Fordtran (Philadelphia: W. B. Saunders Company, 1978), pp. 840–860.

3. Ibid.

4. Isenberg and others, "Pathogenesis of Peptic Ulcer."

5. Charles T. Richardson, "Gastric Ulcer," in *Gastrointestinal Disease*, 2nd ed., eds. Marvin H. Sleisenger and John S. Fordtran (Philadelphia: W. B. Saunders Company, 1978), pp. 875–891.

6. Sturdevant and Walsh, "Duodenal Ulcer."

7. Joseph P. Belber, "Gastroscopy and Duodenoscopy," in *Gastrointestinal Disease*, 2nd ed., eds. Marvin H. Sleisenger and John S. Fordtran (Philadelphia: W. B. Saunders Company, 1978), pp. 691–713.

8. Richardson, "Gastric Ulcer."

9. Walter L. Petersen and John S. Fordtran, "Reduction of Gastric Acidity," in *Gastrointestinal Disease*, 2nd ed., eds. Marvin H. Sleisenger and John S. Fordtran (Philadelphia: W. B. Saunders Company, 1978), pp. 891–913.

10. Ibid.
11. Fordtran, J. S., Morawski, S. G. and Richardson, C. T. In vivo and in vitro evaluation of liquid antacids. *New Eng. J. Med.* 288: 923, 1973.
12. Petersen and Fordtran, "Reduction of Gastric Acidity."
13. Ibid.
14. Ibid.
15. Ibid.
16. James W. Freston, "Cimetidine. I. Developments, Pharmacology, and Efficacy," *Ann. Int. Med.* 97 (1982), 573–580.
17. James W. Freston, "Cimetidine. II. Adverse Reactions and Patterns of Use," *Ann. Int. Med.* 97 (1982) 728–734.
18. Ibid.
19. Freston and Cimetidine, "Developments, Pharmacology, and Efficacy."
20. Charles O. Walker, "Complications of Peptic Ulcer Disease and Indications for Surgery," in *Gastrointestinal Disease,* 2nd ed., eds. Marvin H. Sleisenger and John S. Fordtran (Philadelphia: W. B. Saunders Company, 1978), pp. 914–932.
21. Ibid.
22. James H. Meyer, "Chronic Morbidity after Ulcer Surgery," in *Gastrointestinal Disease,* 2nd ed., eds. Marvin H. Sleisenger and John S. Fordtran (Philadelphia: W. B. Saunders Company, 1978), pp. 947–969.
23. Edward Passaro, Jr. and Bruce Stabile, "Postoperative Recurrent Ulcer," in *Gastrointestinal Disease,* 2nd ed., eds. Marvin H. Sleisenger and John S. Fordtran (Philadelphia: W. B. Saunders Company, 1978), pp. 969–978.

Chapter 3

1. Charles E. Pope, II, "Symptoms of Esophageal Disease," in *Gastrointestinal Disease,* 2nd ed., eds. Marvin H.

Sleisenger and John S. Fordtran (Philadelphbia: W. B. Saunders Company, 1978), pp. 196–199.

2. James L. A. Roth, "Symptomatology Other Than Pain and Discomfort," in *Gastroenterology*, 3rd ed., ed. Henry L. Bockus (Philadelphia: W. B. Saunders Company, 1974), pp. 71–102.

3. Charles E. Pope, II, "Gastroesophageal Reflux Disease (Reflux Esophagitis)," in *Gastrointestinal Disease*, 2nd. ed., eds. Marvin H. Sleisenger and John S. Fordtran (Philadelphia: W. B. Saunders Company, 1978), pp. 541–568.

4. Ibid.

5. Pope, "Symptoms of Esophageal Disease."

6. Roth, "Symptomatology Other Than Pain and Discomfort."

7. Pope, "Gastroesophageal Reflux Disease."

8. Henry L. Bockus, "Diaphragmatic Hernia, Esophageal Hiatus Hernia, Eventration and Paralysis of the Diaphragm," in *Gastroenterology*, 3rd ed., ed. Henry L. Bockus (Philadelphia: W. B. Saunders Company, 1974), pp. 349–374.

9. Ibid.

10. James L. A. Roth, "Reflux Esophagitis and Esophageal Ulcer," in *Gastroenterology*, 3rd ed., ed. Henry L. Bockus (Philadelphia: W. B. Saunders Company, 1974), pp. 247–288.

11. Pope, "Gastroesophageal Reflux Disease."

12. Roth, "Reflux Esophagitis and Esophageal Ulcer."

Chapter 4

1. Michael D. Levitt and John H. Bond, "Intestinal Gas," in *Gastrointestinal Disease*, 2nd. ed., eds. Marvin H. Sleisenger and John S. Fordtran (Philadelphia: W. B. Saunders Company, 1978), pp. 387–393.

2. R. B. Lasser, J. H. Bond, and M. D. Levitt, "The role of intestinal gas in functional abdominal pain," *New Eng. J. Med.* 293 (1975), 524.
3. J. Weiss, "Etiology and Management of Intestinal Gas," *Current Therapy Research* 16 (1974), 909.
4. Levitt and Bond, "Intestinal Gas."

Chapter 5

1. Ghislain Devroede, "Constipation: Mechanisms and Management," in *Gastrointestinal Disease*, 2nd ed., eds. Marvin H. Sleisenger and John S. Fordtran (Philadelphia: W. B. Saunders Company, 1978), pp. 368–386.
2. Ibid.
3. N. Heilburn and C. Bernstein, "Roentgen abnormalities of the large bowel and small intestine associated with prolonged cathartic ingestion," *Radiology* 65 (1955), 549.
4. David Earnest, "Other Diseases of the Colon and Rectum," in *Gastrointestinal Disease*, 2nd. ed., eds. Marvin H. Sleisenger and John S. Fordtran (Philadelphia: W. B. Saunders Company, 1978), pp. 1834–1874.
5. Devroede, "Constipation: Mechanisms and Management."
6. J. Higginson "Etiological factors in gastrointestinal cancer," *J. Nat. Cancer Inst.* 37 (1966), 527.
7. E. L. Wynder and T. Shigematsu, "Environmental factors of cancers of the colon and rectum," *Cancer* 20 (1967), 1520.

Chapter 6

1. Peter M. Loeb, "Diverticular Disease of the Colon," in *Gastrointestinal Disease*, 2nd ed., eds. Marvin H. Sleisenger and John S. Fordtran (Philadelphia: W. B. Saunders Company, 1978), pp. 1745–1771.

2. Ibid.

3. N. S. Painter, and D. P. Burkitt, "Diverticular disease of the colon, a 20th century problem," *Clin. Gastoent.* 4(1975), 3.

4. A. M. Lubbe, "Dietary Evaluation," in "A Comparative Study of Rural and Urban Venda Males," eds. A. L. Van der Merve and S. A. Fellingham, *S. Afr. Med. J.* 45 (1971), 1289.

5. J. H. Cummings, "Progress Report: Dietary Fibre," *Gut* 14(1973), 69.

6. H. Trowell, "Definition of dietary fiber and hypothesis that it is a protective factor in certain diseases," *Amer. J. Clin. Nutr.* 29, (1976), 417.

7. Loeb, "Diverticular Disease of the Colon."

8. H. L. Bockus, "Simple Constipation," in *Gastroenterology*, 3rd. ed., ed. Henry L. Bockus (Philadelphia:W. B. Saunders Company, 1974), pp. 936–953.

9. Loeb, "Diverticular Disease of the Colon."

10. Ibid.

11. Ibid.

12. T. G. Parks, "Surgery of Diverticular Disease of the Colon," in *Gastroenterology,* 3rd ed., ed. Henry L. Bockus (Philadelphia: W. B. Saunders Company, 1974), pp. 1001–1008.

Chapter 7

1. Thomas P. Almy, "Irritable Bowel Syndrome," in *Gastrointestinal Disease*, 2nd ed., eds. Marvin H. Sleisenger and John S. Fordtran (Philadelphia: W. B. Saunders Company, 1978), pp. 1585–1597.

2. T. P. Almy, "Digestive disease as a national problem. II." A white paper by the American Gastroenterology Association. *Gastroenterology* 53 (1967), 821.

3. Almy, "Irritable Bowel Syndrome."

4. William S. Haubrich, "Functional Bowel Disorders," in *Gastroenterology*, 3rd ed., ed. Henry L. Bockus

(Philadelphia: W. B. Saunders Company, 1974), pp. 895–917.

5. H. Dvorkin, F. J. Biel, and T. E. Machella, "Supradiaphragmatic reference of pain from the colon," *Gastroenterology* 22 (1967), 222.
6. Almy, "Irritable Bowel Syndrome."
7. Haubrich, "Functional Bowel Disorders."

Chapter 8

1. Robert M. Donaldson, Jr., "Carbohydrate Intolerance," in *Gastrointestinal Disease*, 2nd ed., eds. Marvin H. Sleisenger and John S. Fordtran (Philadelphia: W. B. Saunders Company, 1978), pp. 1181–1190.
2. Ibid.
3. Gary M. Gray, "Intestinal disaccharidase deficiencies and glucose-galactose malabsorption," in *The Metabolic Basis of Inherited Diseases*, 4th ed., eds. J. B. Stanbury, J. B. Wyngaerden, and D. S. Fredrickson (New York: McGraw-Hill, 1977), Chapter 66.
4. Donaldson, "Carbohydrate Intolerance."
5. Gray, "Intestinal disaccharidase deficiencies . . ."
6. Donaldson, "Carbohydrate Intolerance."
7. Gray, "Intestinal disaccharidase deficiencies . . ."
8. T. M. Bayless, B. Rothfeld, C. Massa, and others, "Lactose and Milk Intolerance: Clinical Implications," *New Eng. J. Med.* 292 (1975), 1156.
9. E. Weser, W. Rubin, I. Ross, and others, "Lactase deficiency in patients with 'irritable bowel syndrome'," *New Eng. J. Med.* 273 (1965), 1070.
10. Donaldson, "Carbohydrate Intolerance."
11. Ibid.

Chapter 9

1. Guenter J. Krejs and John S. Fordtran, "Diarrhea," in *Gastrointestinal Disease*, 2nd ed., eds. Marvin H. Sleisenger and John S. Fordtran (Philadelphia: W. B. Saunders Company, 1978), pp. 313–335.
2. William S. Haubrich, "Traveler's Diarrhea," in *Gastroenterology*, 3rd ed., ed. Henry L. Bockus (Philadelphia: W. B. Saunders Company, 1974), pp. 933–936.
3. Sherwood L. Gorbach, "Traveler's Diarrhea," *New Eng. J. Med.* 307 (1982), 881.
4. H. L. DuPont, P. Sullivan, L. K. Pickering, et al., "Symptomatic treatment of diarrhea with bismuth subsalicylate among students attending a Mexican university," *Gastroenterology* 73 (1977), 715.
5. H. L. DuPont, R. R. Reves, E. Galindo, et al., "Treatment of Traveler's Diarrhea with Trimethoprim/ Sulfamethoxazole and Trimethoprim Alone," *New Eng. J. Med.* 307 (1982), 841.
6. Haubrich, "Traveler's Diarrhea."
7. Lloyd L. Brandborg, "Other Infections, Inflammatory, and Miscellaneous Diseases," in *Gastrointestinal Disease*, 2nd. ed., eds. Marvin H. Sleisenger and John S. Fordtran (Philadelphia: W. B. Saunders Company, 1978), pp. 1076–1093.
8. Kimberly J. Curtis and Marvin H. Sleisenger, "Infections and Parasitic Diseases," in *Gastroenintestinal Disease*, 2nd ed., eds. Marvin H. Sleisenger and John S. Fordtran (Philadelphia: W. B. Saunders Company, 1978), pp. 1679–1715.
9. Ibid.
10. Brandborg, "Other Infections, Inflammatory, and Miscellaneous Diseases."

11. Martin J. Blaser and L. Barth Reller, "Campylobacter enteritis," *New Eng. J. Med.* 305 (1981), 1444.
12. Brandborg, "Other Infections, Inflammatory, and Miscellaneous Diseases."
13. Lloyd L. Brandborg, "Parasitic Diseases," in *Gastrointestinal Disease*, 2nd ed., eds. Marvin H. Sleisenger and John H. Fordtran (Philadelphia: W. B. Saunders Company, 1978), pp. 1154–1181.

Chapter 10

1. Theodore R. Schrock, "Diseases of Anorectum," in *Gastrointestinal Disease,* 2nd. ed., eds. Marvin H. Sleisenger and John S. Fordtran (Philadelphia: W. B. Saunders Company, 1978), pp. 1875–1889.
2. P. R. Hawley, "Hemorrhoids," *Recent Advan. Surg.* 8 (1973), 235.
3. Schrock, "Diseases of the Anorectum."
4. Ibid.
5. Ibid.

Chapter 11

1. N. G. Kock, "A New Look at Ileostomy," *Surg. Ann.* 8 (1976), 241.
2. Ibid.

Chapter 12

1. Joseph B. Kirsner and Ray G. Shorter, "Recent Developments in 'Nonspecific' Inflammatory Bowel Disease, Part One," *New Eng. J. Med.* 306 (1982), 775.
2. Joseph B. Kirsner and Ray G. Shorter, "Recent Developments in 'Nonspecific' Inflammatory Bowel Disease, Part II," *New Eng. J. Med.* 306 (1982), 837.
3. Ibid.

4. F. C. Edwards and S. C. Truelove, "The Course and Prognosis of Ulcerative Colitis. II. Long-term Prognosis," *Gut* 4 (1964), 309.

5. John P. Cello and James H. Meyer, "Ulcerative Colitis," in *Gastrointestinal Disease*, 2nd. ed., eds. Marvin H. Sleisenger and John S. Fordtran (Philadelphia: W. B. Saunders Company, 1978), pp. 1597–1653.

6. F. C. Edwards and S. C. Truelove, "The Course and Prognosis of Ulcerative Colitis. I. Short-term Prognosis," *Gut* 4 (1964), 299.

7. Kirsner and Shorter, "Recent Developments in 'Nonspecific' Inflammatory Bowel Disease."

8. J. J. Misiewicz, J. E. Lennard-Jones, A. M. Connell, and others, "Controlled Trial of Sulphasalazine in Maintenance Therapy for Ulcerative Colitis," *Lancet* I (1965), 185.

9. Kirsner and Shorter, "Recent Developments in 'Nonspecific' Inflammatory Bowel Disease."

10. W. R. Thayer, Jr., "Malignancy in Inflammatory Bowel Disease," in *Inflammatory Bowel Disease*, 2nd. ed., eds. Joseph B. Kirsner and Ray G. Shorter (Philadelphia: Lea and Febiger, 1980), pp. 265–278.

11. R. H. Riddell and B. C. Morson, "Value of Sigmoidoscopy and Biopsy in Detection of Carcinoma and Premalignant Change in Ulcerative Colitis and Crohn's Disease," *Gut* 20 (1979), 575.

12. Kirsner and Shorter, "Recent Developments in 'Nonspecific' Inflammatory Bowel Disease."

13. Victor W. Fazio, "Toxic Megacolon in Ulcerative Colitis and Crohn's Disease," in *Clinics in Gastroenterology May 1980*, ed. Richard G. Farmer (Philadelphia: W. B. Saunders Company, 1980), pp. 389–407.

Chapter 13

1. B. B. Crohn, "Granulomatous Disease of the Large and Small Bowel. A Historical Survey," *Gastroenterology* 52 (1967), 767.

2. Robert M. Donaldson, Jr., "Crohn's Disease of the Small Bowel," in *Gastrointestinal Disease,* 2nd ed., eds. Marvin H. Sleisenger and John S. Fordtran (Philadelphia: W. B. Saunders Company, 1978), pp. 1052–1076.

3. Joseph B. Kirsner and Ray G. Shorter, "Recent Developments in 'Nonspecific' Inflammatory Bowel Disease, Part One," *New Eng. J. Med.* 306 (1982), 775.

4. Albert I. Mendoloff, "The Epidemiology of Inflammatory Bowel Disease," in *Clinics of Gastroenterology, May 1980,* ed. Richard G. Farmer (Philadelphia: W. B. Saunders, Co., 1980), pp. 259–270.

5. Richard G. Farmer, W. A. Hawk, R. B. Turnbell, and others, "Clinicopathy with Comparison of Transmural Colitis and Ulcerative Colitis," *Modern Medicine,* June 12, 1972, pp. 94–99.

6. Kirsner and Shorter, "Recent Developments."

7. Burton I. Korelitz, "Carcinoma of the Intestinal Tract in Crohn's Disease: Results of a Survey Conducted by the National Foundation for Ileitis and Colitis," *American Journal of Gastroenterology* 78 (1983), p. 44.

8. A. J. Greenstein, D. B. Sachar, and B. S. Pasternack, "Re-operation and Recurrence in Crohn's Colitis and Ileocolitis," *New England Journal of Medcicine* 293 (1975), 685.

9. M. R. Lock, R. G. Farmer, and V. W. Fazio, "Recurrence and Re-operation for Crohn's Disease," *New England Journal of Medicine* 304 (1981), 1586.

10. R. W. Summers, D. M. Switz, J. R. Sessions, Jr., and others, "National Cooperative Crohn's Disease Study: Results of Drug Treatment," *Gastroenterology* 77 (1979), 847.

Chapter 14

1. R. S. Stubbs, R. F. McLoy, and L. H. Blumgart, "Cholelithiasis and Cholecystitis Surgical Treatment," in *Clinics in Gastroenterology,* January 1983, eds. Meinhard

Classen and Hans W. Schreiber (Philadelphia: W. B. Saunders Co., 1983), pp. 179–201.

2. Boston Collaborative Drug Surveillance Program Report, "Oral Contraceptives and Venous Thromboemboli Disease, Surgically Confirmed Gallbladder Disease and Heart Tumors," *Lancet Journal* 1399 (1973).
3. Henry L. Backus, "Cholelithiasis. Part II. Clinical Aspects," in *Gastroenterology*, 3rd ed., ed. Henry L. Backus (Philadelphia: W. B. Saunders Co., 1974), pp. 752–785.
4. W. P. Mikkalsen, "The pathogenesis and management of acute cholecystitis," *Nebr. Med. J.* 55 (1979), 20.
5. Y. Edlund, J. Eldh, and N. G. Kock, "Bacteriologic investigations of the biliary system and liver in biliary tract disease correlated to clinical data and microstructure of the gallbladder and liver," *Acta. Chir. Scand.* 116 (1958), 461.
6. Lawrence W. Way and Marvin H. Sleisenger, "Cholelithiasis and chronic cholecystitis," *Gastrointestinal Disease* (1978), pp. 1294–1302.
7. J. Edward Beck and Allan A. Kaplan, "Choledocholithiasis," in *Gastroenterology* (1974), pp. 843–864.
8. L. Safrany, "Endoscopic treatment of biliary tract disease. An International Study," *Lancet* 2 (1978), 983.
9. J. L. Thistle, A. F. Hofmann, and B. J. Oh, "Chemotherapy for Gallstone Dissolution," *JAMA* 239 (1978), 1041.

Chapter 15

1. J. T. Danzi, "A Clinical Approach to the Diagnosis of Pancreatic Disease and a Diagnostic Approach to the Icteric Patient," *The Gutherie Bulletin* 48 (1979), 195.
2. H. Sarles and A. Gerolami-Santandria, "Chronic pancreatitis," *Clin. Gastroent.* 1 (1972), 167.
3. N. Darle, G. Lebrenil, Y. Edlund, "Ultrastructure of the rat exocrine pancreas after long-term intake of ethanol," *Gastroenterology* 58 (1970), 62.

4. L. Way, T. Gadacz, and L. Goldman, "Surgical treatment of chronic pancreatitis," *Amer. J. Surg.* 127 (1974), 202.

5. J. H. Ransom, K. M. Rifkind, and J. W. Turner, "Prognostic signs and non-operative peritoneal lavage in acute pancreatitis," *Surg. Gynec. Obstet.* 193 (1978), 209.

6. I. Fras, E. Litin, and L. Bartholomew, "Mental symptoms as an aid in the early diagnosis of cancer of the pancreas," *Gastroenterology* 55 (1968), 191.

Chapter 16

1. R. A. Garibaldi, B. Hanson, and M. B. Gregg, "Impact of illicit drug-associated hepatitis on viral hepatitis morbidity reports in United States," *J. Infect. Dis.* 126 (1972), 288.

2. D. E. Dietzman, J. P. Harnisch, C. G. Ray, and others, "Hepatitis B surface antigen and antibody. Prevalence in homosexual and heterosexual men," *JAMA* 238 (1977), 2625.

3. R. Aach and R. Kahn, "Post-transfusion hepatitis: Current Perspectives," *Ann. Intern. Med.* 92 (1980), 539.

4. D. P. Francis and J. E. Maynard, "The transmission and outcome of hepatitis A, B and non-A, non-B: A review," *Epidemiol. Rev.* 1 (1979), 17.

5. Recommendations of the Immunization Practices Advisory Committee. Department of Health and Human Services: Immune Globulin for Protection Against Viral Hepatitis. *Ann. Intern. Med.* 96 (1982), 193.

6. S. Krugman, "The newly licensed hepatitis B vaccine: Characteristics and indications for use," *JAMA* 247 (1982), 2012.

Chapter 17

1. A. M. Hoyumpa, P. V. Desmond, G. R. Avant, and others, "Hepatic encephalopathy," *Gastroenterology* 76 (1979), 184.

2. H. O. Conn, W. W. Lindenmuth, C. J. May, and others, "Prophylactic portocaval shunts," *Medicine* 51 (1972), 27.

3. P. Y. Wong, G. C. McCoy, A. Spielberg, and others, "The hepatorenal syndrome," *Gastroenterology* 77 (1979), 1326.

4. W. Szmuneness, "Hepatocellular carcinoma and the hepatitis B virus: Evidence of a causal association," *Prog. Med. Virol.* 24 (1978), 40.

5. S. Krugman, "The newly licensed hepatitis B vaccine: Characteristics and indications for use," *JAMA* 247 (1982), 2012.

Chapter 18

1. Lloyd L. Brandborg, "Neoplastic Disease of the Alimentary Tract," in *Cecil Text Books of Medicine*, 15th ed., eds. Paul B. Beeson, Walsh McDermott, and James B. Wyngaarden (Philadelphia: W. B. Saunders Co., 1979), pp. 1596–1597.

2. Thomas F. O'Brien, "Neoplasms of the Large Intestine," in *Cecil Text Books of Medicine*, 15th ed., eds. Paul B. Beeson, Walsh McDermott, and James B. Wyngaarden (Philadelphia: W. B. Saunders Co., 1979), pp. 1606–1610.

3. W. J. Burdette, *Carcinoma of Colon and Antecedent Epithelium* (Springfield, Ill.: Charles C Thomas, 1970).

4. R. Scott Jones and Marvin H. Sleisenger, "Cancer of the Colon and Rectum," in *Gastrointestinal Disease*, 2nd ed., eds. Marvin H. Sleisenger and John S. Fordtran (Philadelphia: W. B. Saunders Company, 1978), pp. 1784–1800.

5. Ibid.

6. E. M. Copeland, L. D. Miller, and R. J. Jones, "Prognostic Factors in Carcinoma of the Colon and Rectum," *Amer. J. Surg.* 116 (1968), 875.

7. Brandborg, "Neoplastic Disease."

8. Ibid.

9. G. McNeer and G. T. Pauls, *Neoplasms of the Stomach* (Philadelphia: J. B. Lippincott Co., 1967).
10. Lloyd L. Brandborg, "Polyps, Tumors and Cancer of the Stomach," in *GID* (1978), pp. 752–776.
11. N. Zamcheck, E. Grable, A. B. Ley, and others, "Occurrence of Gastric Cancer Among Patients with Pernicious Anemia of the Boston City Hospital," *New Eng. J. Med.* 252 (1955), 1103.
12. Brandborg, "Polyps, Tumors and Cancer of the Stomach."

Chapter 19

1. John Q. Stauffer, "Polypoid Tumors of the Colon," in *Gastrointestinal Disease,* 2nd ed., eds. Marvin H. Sleisenger and John S. Fordtran (Philadelphia: W. B. Saunders Company, 1978), pp. 1771–1784.
2. T. Muto, H. J. R. Bussey, and B. Morson, "The evolution of cancer of the colon and rectum," *Cancer* 36 (1975), 2251.
3. W. I. Wolff and H. Shiniga, "Endoscopic polypectomy," *Cancer* 36 (1975), 683.

Index